Curbside
Consultation
of the ACL

49 Clinical Questions

CURBSIDE CONSULTATION IN ORTHOPEDICS
SERIES

SERIES EDITOR, BERNARD R. BACH, JR., MD

Curbside
Consultation
of the ACL
49 Clinical Questions

Bernard R. Bach, Jr., MD
Director, Division of Sports Medicine
Claude Lambert-Susan Thomson Professor of Orthopedic Surgery
RUSH University Medical Center
Midwest Orthopaedics at RUSH
Chicago, IL

and

Nikhil N. Verma, MD
Assistant Professor, Division of Sports Medicine
Department of Orthopaedic Surgery
RUSH University Medical Center
Midwest Orthopaedics at RUSH
Chicago, IL

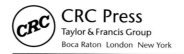

CRC Press
Taylor & Francis Group
Boca Raton London New York

CRC Press is an imprint of the
Taylor & Francis Group, an **informa** business

Delivering the best in health care information and education worldwide

First published 2008 by SLACK Incorporated

Published 2024 by CRC Press
2385 NW Executive Center Drive, Suite 320, Boca Raton FL 33431

and by CRC Press
4 Park Square, Milton Park, Abingdon, Oxon, OX14 4RN

CRC Press is an imprint of Taylor & Francis Group, LLC

© 2008 Taylor & Francis Group

Library of Congress Cataloging-in-Publication Data

Curbside consultation of the ACL : 49 clinical questions / [edited by] Bernard R. Bach, Jr. and Nikhil N. Verma.
    p. ; cm.
  Includes bibliographical references and index.
  ISBN-13: 978-1-55642-825-8 (alk. paper)
  ISBN-10: 1-55642-825-1 (alk. paper)
  1. Anterior cruciate ligament--Surgery--Miscellanea. I. Bach, Bernard R. II. Verma, Nikhil N.
  [DNLM: 1. Anterior Cruciate Ligament--injuries. 2. Anterior Cruciate Ligament--surgery. 3. Athletic Injuries--surgery. 4. Reconstructive Surgical Procedures--methods. WE 870 C9756 2008]

RD561.C824 2008
617.4'7--dc22

                              2008000125

  ISBN: 9781556428258 (pbk)
  ISBN: 9781003523727 (ebk)

  DOI: 10.1201/9781003523727

Dedication

This book is dedicated to my parents, Bernard and Dorothea Bach, for their guidance, nurturing, parenting, and sacrifices; to my wife, Elizabeth, and children, David and Laura, who are the joys of my life, and to my extended family—my sports partners at RUSH, the residents, and sports medicine fellows that I have mentored.

— BRB

To my parents; without their support, I would not be where I am today. And to my wife, Shaila, and to Neil and Jay; without their sacrifices today, I would not have the opportunities of tomorrow.

— NNV

Contents

Acknowledgments

We gratefully acknowledge the outstanding efforts of the staff at SLACK Incorporated in helping bring *Curbside Consultation of the ACL: 49 Clinical Questions* to fruition. From the conceptual development to the completion of the final product, the Slack staff has done an outstanding job. Special kudos to Carrie Kotlar, who played a major role in the early developmental stages; Kim Shigo and Suzanne Miduski in the editorial and pre-publishing stages; and John Bond, Vice President and Publisher at SLACK. We are extremely appreciative of the efforts and professionalism that made this project enjoyable and easier than it might have been. Thanks SLACK!

About the Editors

Bernard R. Bach, Jr., MD, graduated form Harvard College in 1975, the University of Cincinnati College of Medicine in 1979, and obtained general surgery and orthopaedic training at the New England Deaconess Hospital (1979 to 1981) and Combined Harvard Orthopedic Residency program (1981 to 1985) respectively. He completed a Sports Medicine and Shoulder Fellowship at the Hospital for Special Surgery in 1986. At RUSH University Medical Center in Chicago, Bach is currently the Claude N. Lambert-Helen S. Thomson Professor of Orthopaedic Surgery, the director of the Division of Sports Medicine, and has been the RUSH Sports Medicine Fellowship director since 1988. Dr. Bach has published over 400 peer-reviewed manuscripts, abstracts, books, chapters, guest edited monographs, and internet publications. He has served as president of the Harvard Quigley Sports Medicine Society (2003), the Herodicus Society (2005 to 2006), and the American Orthopedic Society for Sports Medicine (2007 to 2008). He is a member of the Illinois Athletic Trainers' Hall of Fame and has served on the board of directors for the Illinois Special Olympics, the Orthopedic Research and Education Foundation, and the American Orthopedic Society for Sports Medicine. Dr. Bach assists with the care of professional athletes as one of the team physicians for the Chicago White Sox and Chicago Bulls.

Nikhil N. Verma, MD, graduated form the University of Michigan in 1994, the University of Pennsylvania School of Medicine in 1998, and completed his surgical internship and orthopedic residency at Rush University Medical Center (1998 to 2003). He completed a Sports Medicine and Shoulder Fellowship at the Hospital for Special Surgery in 2004 before returning to join the staff of the Department of Orthopedics, Section of Sports Medicine, at Rush University Medical Center as an assistant professor. Dr. Verma currently serves as a member of the American Orthopaedic Society for Sports Medicine self-assessment committee and is a member of the editorial board for the Arthroscopy journal. He has coauthored multiple technique and review articles, book chapters, and peer-reviewed manuscripts in the field of sports medicine. Additionally, he has served as a faculty member for both national and international courses in arthroscopic surgery of the shoulder, elbow, and knee. He serves as head orthopedic team physician for the Chicago Bandits and Chicago Force as well as multiple high school teams in the Chicago metro area. Dr. Verma assists with the care of professional athletes as one of the team physicians for the Chicago White Sox and Chicago Bulls.

Contributing Authors

Answorth A. Allen, MD
Associate Attending Orthopaedic Surgeon
Hospital for Special Surgery
Associate Professor, Orthopaedic Surgery
Weill Medical College of Cornell University
New York, NY

Annunziato Amendola, MD
University of Iowa
Iowa City, IA

Stephen F. Brockmeier, MD
Perry Orthopedics and Sports Medicine
Charlotte, NC

Robert H. Brophy, MD
Washington University School of Medicine
St. Louis, MO

Matthew Busam, MD
Cincinnati Sports Medicine
Cincinnati, OH

Charles A. Bush-Joseph, MD
Professor of Orthopaedic Surgery
RUSH University Medical Center
Managing Member, Midwest Orthopaedics at
RUSH
Chicago, IL

James L. Carey, MD
Assistant Professor of Orthopaedics and
Rehabilitation, Vanderbilt Sports Medicine
Vanderbilt University Medical Center
Nashville, TN

Brian J. Cole, MD, MBA
Professor of Orthopedic Surgery
RUSH University Medical Center
Chicago, IL

Anne E. Colton, MD
Surgical Orthopaedic Associates
Broomall, PA

Jerome J. DaSilva, MD
Sports Medicine Fellow Rush University
Medical Center
Chicago, IL

Warren R. Dunn, MD, MPH
Assistant Professor, Orthopaedics &
Rehabilitation
Vanderbilt Sports Medicine Center
Assistant Professor, Medicine & Public Health
Center for Health Services Research
Team Physician Vanderbilt University
Nashville, TN

Nicholas T. Dutcheshen, MD
Massachusettes General Hospital/Harvard
Medical School
Department of Sports Medicine
Boston, MA

James D. Ferrari, MD
Advanced Orthopedics and Sports Medicine
Specialists
Denver, CO

Kyle R. Flik, MD
Sports Medicine
Northeast Orthopaedics, LLP
Albany, NY

Seth C. Gamradt, MD
UCLA Department of Orthopaedic Surgery
Los Angeles, CA

Thomas J. Gill, MD
Massachusettes General Hospital/Harvard
Medical School
Director, Department of Sports Medicine
Boston, MA

R. Edward Glenn, Jr., MD
Tennessee Orthopaedic Alliance
Nachville, TN

Contributing Authors

Brian Kerr, MD
Private Practice
Traverse City, MI

Aimee S. Klapach, MD
Sports & Orthopaedic Specialists
Edina, Minnesota

John D. MacGillivray, MD
Assistant Professor of Orthopedic Surgery
Weill Medical College of Cornell University
Assistant Attending Orthopedic Surgeon
Hospital for Special Surgery
New York, NY

Eric C. McCarty, MD
University of Colorado School of Medicine
Denver, CO

L. Pearce McCarty, III, MD
Sports and Orthopaedic Specialists, P.A.
Edina, MN

Shane J. Nho, MD, MS
Resident, Department of Orthopedic Surgery
Weill Medical College of Cornell University
Hospital for Special Surgery
New York, NY

Luke S. Oh, MD
Chief Resident of Orthopaedic Surgery
Hospital for Special Surgery
New York, NY

Michael Pensak, BS
Medical Student
SUNY Downstate College of Medicine
Brooklyn, NY

Matthew T. Provencher, MD, LCDR, MC, USN
Department of Orthopaedic Surgery
Division of Orthopaedic Shoulder, Knee, and
Sports Surgery
Naval Medical Center San Diego
San Diego, CA

Scott A. Rodeo, MD
Professor of Orthopaedic Surgery
The Hospital for Special Surgery
New York, NY

John-Paul H. Rue, MD, LCDR, MC, USN
Department of Orthopaedic Surgery
National Naval Medical Center
Bethesda, Maryland

Kurt P. Spindler, MD
Vanderbilt University
Nashville, TN

Thomas L. Wickiewicz, MD
Attending Orthopaedic Surgeon
Sports Medicine and Shoulder Service
Hospital for Special Surgery
New York, NY

Riley J. Williams, III, MD
Hospital for Special Surgery
New York, NY

Preface

One might ask, "Why another sports medicine text?" As an orthopedic resident in the early 1980s, there was a paucity of orthopedic texts in general, and certainly very few in sports medicine. At that time, sports medicine was a fledgling field. Today, orthopedic sports medicine is one of the most popular subspecialties within the field of orthopedic surgery. One in four graduating orthopedic residents pursues postgraduate training in sports medicine. Last year at RUSH University Medical Center, we had over 150 applications for our sports medicine fellowship! For those individuals preparing to take part II of the American Board of Orthopedic Surgery oral examinations, a review of applicants' surgical case logs demonstrated that sports/arthroscopically related surgical procedures comprised five of the eight most commonly performed surgical procedures. Anterior cruciate ligament (ACL) reconstruction procedures were overall the sixth most commonly performed procedures performed among these young orthopedic surgeons. There is currently a plethora of sports medicine and knee related textbooks. Most of these texts are all encompassing. Few are focused, topic specific textbooks.

Many textbooks concentrate on technique specifics. Certainly many of the chapters the senior author (BRB) has contributed to textbooks have dealt with the subtle nuances of ACL reconstruction techniques. While there has been a push towards Level I prospective randomized clinical trials to answer many pertinent questions in orthopedics and sports medicine, the sage advice of an experienced expert is still warranted. Why else would we have grand rounds speakers, visiting professors, keynote speakers, symposiae, and point–counterpoint debates at our meetings? *Curbside Consultation in the ACL: 49 Clinical Questions* is an attempt to model after my evolutionary experience attending postgraduate continuing medical education meetings. As I (BRB) have evolved from a meeting attendee to a frequent faculty person, a committee member, and now in a position of leadership as President (2007 to 2008) of the American Orthopedic Society for Sports Medicine, much of my current learning is no longer done in the lecture hall but in the foyers picking the brains of my colleagues. I usually attend meetings with specific goals in mind. I have specific questions that I need answered. These are called "curbside consults," much like when we walk down the halls of the hospital and a colleague stops you and asks your opinion on a topic or problem.

Curbside Consultation in the ACL: 49 Clinical Questions is not an all encompassing authoritative text dealing with the ACL. As you peruse the table of contents, it is striking to note the focused questions that deal with many of our current concerns, concepts, and controversies. This text is directed to residents, fellows, and general orthopedic surgeons who perform ACL surgery. This 180 page plus text is inexpensive, focused, easily readable, and digestible. It assumes a core knowledge in orthopedic sports medicine and the ACL. The 49 chapters are divided into short "to the point" discussions of important fundamentals balanced with current controversies. The book is divided into six sections: preoperative, intraoperative, postoperative, failed ACL, pediatric and adolescent ACL, and miscellaneous ACL issues. This is the type of text that you could study over a weekend as each "chapter" is a no nonsense two to four page discussion of the specific topic. Trust me—if you read this text, you will have a finger on the pulse of ACL issues in 2008!

Dr. Verma and I are grateful to our contributing authors who have shared their expertise for this textbook. In fact, I have frequently "curbsided" many of these colleagues and received sage advice. We hope that this textbook becomes a well-worn threadbare reference in your library!

Bernard R. Bach, Jr., MD
January 4, 2008

Foreword

When Dr. Bach asked me to write a foreword to this new text, I was intrigued by the format. This approach to learning allows the learner to choose what aspects of the topic he or she wishes to consider. This format becomes an interactive activity, which engages the learner and provides the opportunity to have a comprehensive appraisal of anterior cruciate ligament (ACL) reconstruction or to select an individual curriculum for learning.

This text by a group of experts offers an evolution to the approach to ACL treatment in the changing environment as seen over the last 25 years. In 1902, Sir William Osler said the philosophies of one age have become the absurdities of the next and the foolishness of yesterday has become the wisdom of tomorrow. The use of soft tissue grafts and allografts, the approach to tunnel placement, and the aggressive return of motion reflect the enormous change that has occurred over the past 25 years. It was impossible to do single incision endoscopic reconstruction 30 years ago, and nowadays it is commonplace and, in fact, the standard of care.

The value of this monograph on a focused topic is its comprehensive nature, the credibility of the editors, and the excellent manner in which the material is organized. The senior author has been known for a pragmatic approach to ACL reconstruction as well as the extensive critical analysis he has done of his own results. Such a critical analysis is an essential part of the format in this text as well.

I also find it amazing and a credit to the editors of this book that there is so little redundancy. I would expect with so many authors there would be a good deal of repetition and yet in these presentations there is very little overlap, and that is a credit to the editors for the manner in which the material is organized and presented. As someone who has watched ACL reconstruction over the last 30 years, I feel comforted by the answers to these 49 questions. Clearly we have come a long way with our understanding of the evaluation, treatment, and rehabilitation of the ACL injury. This material is a tribute to the understanding of the evolution of ACL reconstruction and the contributions of not only these authors but the many who preceded them. I congratulate the authors and editors, and I recommend this approach for the learner.

William A. Grana, MD, MPH
Professor, Orthopaedic Surgery
University of Arizona
Tucson, AZ

SECTION I

PREOPERATIVE QUESTIONS

WHAT ARE THE INDICATIONS FOR SURGICAL OR NONSURGICAL TREATMENT?

Bernard R. Bach, Jr., MD, and Matthew Busam, MD

Multiple factors impact recommendations for surgery. One consideration is patient age. At one end of the spectrum is the adolescent anterior cruciate ligament (ACL)-deficient patient, and at the other extreme are patients over the age of 40. It has been previously demonstrated that satisfactory outcomes can be achieved in over 80% of patients treated nonoperatively in this older cohort provided that activity modification occurs.[1] In this group rehabilitation is critical. Nevertheless, there are patients who may require surgical treatment. An absolute age is not used as a criterion for determining whether a patient is or is not a candidate for surgical treatment. Approximately 15% of the ACL patients in our practice are over age 40. We take into consideration the activity level, hours of sports per week, and patient expectations.

At the other end of the spectrum are the skeletally immature patients. The ACL-deficient knee in the skeletally immature patient behaves similarly to an adult and is at risk for reinjury, meniscal tears, and chondral injury.[2] In the growing child, there are concerns of future growth, particularly premature growth arrest or angular deformity, that must be considered when determining which, if any, surgical procedure is best. Skeletal age, onset of menarche, Tanner stage, and even the parents' heights are all factors that may be considered. In patients with open growth plates with more than a year and a half of skeletal growth remaining, we recommend a soft-tissue graft (hamstring), using a small vertical tibial tunnel. We place the femoral component of the graft in an over-the-top femoral position without violating the femoral growth plate. In prepubescent athletes, we consider an extra physeal tibial trough.

Activity level plays an extremely important role in consideration of surgery. Sports activity levels can be defined as category I: jumping, pivoting, hard cutting (basketball, football, and soccer); category II: lateral motion but less jumping or hard cutting (baseball, racquet sports, and skiing); and category III: sports with more linear activities (jogging, running, and low-impact sports such as swimming).[3] Occupational levels may play a role as well and are similar to sports levels. Patients who perform heavy manual work and are working at height, or on uneven surfaces, are considered candidates for surgical treatment.[3] Individuals performing light manual work do not, in our opinion, require surgical reconstruction. In individuals such as police officers, firemen, and construction workers, we typically recommend surgical reconstruction.

The athlete's skill level is another consideration. Athletes may be categorized as recreational, interscholastic, intercollegiate, and professional. In general, the more intense the athletic competition, particularly taking into consideration the patient's age and hours of sports per week, ACL reconstruction is recommended.

Sport-specific considerations correlate well with category I and category II sports. In general, patients who participate in football, basketball, volleyball, skiing, soccer, and rugby are, in our opinion, clear-cut candidates for reconstructive surgery.

Associated ligamentous injury may play a factor in recommending surgery as well as in the timing of surgery. ACL injury may occur concurrently with medial collateral ligament involvement. It is critical to recognize that the proximal medial collateral ligament (MCL) injury pattern may be associated with knee stiffness; therefore, full motion should be achieved before recommending ACL treatment. The MCL is typically treated nonoperatively. We rehab the MCL and use a brace for more significant MCL injuries, followed by elective ACL reconstruction. On the other side of the knee, the posterolateral corner may be injured with the ACL or a patient may sustain a bicruciate, that is, ACL/posterial cruciate ligament (PCL) injury. More significant trauma may be involved in bicruciate with collateral ligament injury or knee dislocations. Severe injuries may also be associated with patellar instability and/or patellar tendon rupture. As a generalization, the more severe the injury is, the more likely that ACL reconstruction will be recommended by a surgeon.

The last 20 years have witnessed a trend toward meniscal preservation. It is evident that there are higher failure rates in meniscal repair in the ACL-deficient knee.[4] Some surgeons advocate a single versus staged procedure for meniscal repair with or without ACL reconstruction. It is recognized that lateral meniscal tears occur more commonly acutely, medial meniscal tears occur more commonly in chronic ACL-deficient knees, and the medial meniscus is more frequently associated with a displaced bucket handle tear.[5]

The timing of surgery plays an important role. Acute reconstructions should not be performed unless motion is recovered.[6] We attempt to separate the post-traumatic and postsurgical inflammatory phases by deferring surgery until motion is recovered.

Historically, response to functional ACL bracing was considered a major factor in the determination of surgical versus nonsurgical treatment. Although Noyes[7] popularized the rule of one-thirds (ie, one-third do well, one-third modify activity, and one-third require surgical treatment), perspectives are changing with regards to the use of bracing, and in fact, the majority of patients in our practice desire ACL reconstruction rather than to attempt functional knee bracing. There is little literature to assess how often recurrent instability should be considered as an indication for ACL surgery. It is important to differentiate between major and minor episodes. If someone is complaining of his knee "giving way" nearly every day, multiple times per day, it more likely is meniscal pathology. Major episodes of instability are usually associated with gross giving way and collapsing to the ground. Some surgeons feel that more than 2 major episodes annually are an indication for ACL reconstruction.

Late ACL reconstruction factors include preinjury sports participation, patient age, hours of sports per week, and side-to-side differences on KT-1000 testing. Arthritis and malalignment must be carefully considered; an osteotomy may be the preferred method of treatment with staged ACL reconstruction. In the arthritic patient with pain complaints, ACL reconstruction is less likely to be predictably beneficial. Patients who have more than 5-mm side-to-side translation on KT-1000 and are involved in more than 4 hours of sports per week are at high risk for reinjury, and those that are between 5 and 7 mm but are involved in less than 4 hours of sports per week are at moderate risk for reinjury.[3]

Patient compliance is a major consideration. It is critical to assess the patient's compliance and determine whether he or she is committed to postreconstructive rehabilitation. This may impact the type of graft that is recommended. One needs to assess the patient's goals and determine whether he or she is realistic and consistent with the surgeon's goals and abilities.

Social considerations are also important. We have to consider timing relative to school vacations or relative to the next athletic season. We have seen patients who anticipate job or career changes and may have a change in their health insurance coverage. This may impact their desire to be reconstructed. Furthermore, if they change insurance and have a pre-existing condition, this may impact whether they may be covered on their next health insurance policy. Some patients have presented to our office desiring ACL reconstruction because of future anticipated changes in health care delivery systems, which may make it more difficult to have elective ACL reconstructive surgery. We have seen patients who anticipate leaving their parents' health plan following the conclusion of their college education and desire ACL reconstruction. On occasion, we have had a parent present to the office desiring ACL reconstruction because they want to "play" with their children as they get older. Patients considering starting families may present to our office contemplating ACL reconstruction because of concerns about knee instability during pregnancy.

In summary, surgical considerations for ACL treatment involve high-risk sports, the competitive athlete, recurrent knee instability, and meniscal symptoms. In the acute injury, the activity lifestyle is probably the most important factor, whereas in the chronic ACL-deficient patient, recurrent instability is the most important factor.

References

1. Ciccotti MG, Lombardo SJ, Nonweiler B, Pink W. Nonoperative treatment of ruptures of the anterior cruciate ligament in middle aged patients. *J Bone Joint Surg.* 1994;76-A:1315-1321.
2. Mizuta H, Kubota K, Shiraishi M, Otsuka Y, Nagamota N, Takagi K. The conservative treatment of complete tears of the anterior cruciate ligament in skeletally immature patients. *J Bone Joint Surg.* 1995;77-B:890-894.
3. Daniel DM, Stone ML, Dobson BE, Fithian DC, Rossman DJ, Kaufman KR. Fate of the ACL-injured patient. A prospective outcome study. *Am J Sports Med.* 1994;22(5):632-644.
4. Bach BR Jr, Dennis M, Balin J, Hayden J. Arthroscopic meniscal repair: analysis of treatment failures. *J Knee Surg.* 2005;18:278-284.
5. Bellabarba C, Bush-Joseph CA, Bach BR Jr. Patterns of meniscal injury in the anterior cruciate ligament-deficient knee: a review of the literature. *Am J Orthop.* 1997;26:18-23.
6. Shelbourne KD, Wilckens JH, Mollabashy A, DeCarlo M. Arthrofibrosis in acute anterior cruciate ligament reconstruction. The effect of timing of reconstruction and rehabilitation. *Am J Sports Med.* 1991;19(4):332-336.
7. Noyes FR, Mooar PA, Matthews DS, Butler DL. The symptomatic anterior cruciate deficient knee. Part I: the long term functional disability in athletically active individuals. *J Bone Joint Surg.* 1983;65-A:154-162.

WHAT ARE THE RADIOGRAPHIC, MAGNETIC RESONANCE, AND KT-1000 CHARACTERISTICS OF AN ACL-INJURED KNEE?

Matthew Busam, MD, and Bernard R. Bach, Jr., MD

Physical exam is the most important tool for diagnosing an anterior cruciate ligament (ACL) injury. A positive Lachman test and a demonstrable pivot-shift phenomenon are pathognomonic of ACL deficiency.[1] However, in the setting of pain, the patient may guard significantly enough to prevent a reliable physical exam, particularly with pivot shift testing. In addition, pain from a bone bruise or collateral ligament injury may be difficult to discern from meniscal or osteochondral pathology. Furthermore, many patients present to the orthopedic surgeon already having obtained radiographs and/or a magnetic resonance image (MRI) from their primary care provider or emergency room. The orthopedic surgeon must be skilled in interpreting this information and cannot rely on the radiology report, which may or may not be available. In the setting of an ACL injury, arthrometric and radiographic data are essential tools to assist the clinician in confirming the diagnosis and elucidating the nature of concomitant pathologies.

The KT-1000 arthrometer (Medmetric, San Diego, CA) plays a valuable role in elucidating exact translation and confirming ACL deficiency. The newer KT-2000 differs from its predecessor only in its ability to graphically plot data on x- and y-axes. It measures anterior translation of the tibia on the femur at 15-lb and 20-lb increments and at maximum manual testing (Figure 2-1). The compliance index is the difference between the values at 20 and 15 lbs. The KT-1000 is an instrumented Lachman test. Daniels and associates found side-to-side differences between the normal and the injured knee to be an important marker. A side-to-side difference of 3 mm or more at 20 lbs or maximum manual testing was diagnostic of an ACL disruption.[2] In addition, they recommended that a compliance index of 2 mm to 2.5 mm be considered equivocal for an of ACL injury, while a compliance index of 3 mm or more was diagnostic.[2] In another series, Bach and colleagues

Figure 2-1. Clinical photo of KT-1000 in use.

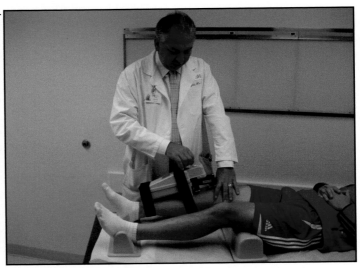

considered translation of 11 mm or more on 20 lbs or maximum manual testing diagnostic of an ACL tear. In addition, they noted that all control subjects had a compliance index of 2 mm or less; therefore, they considered a compliance index of more than 2 mm diagnostic of an ACL tear.[3] In general, a maximum manual side-to-side difference of greater than 3 mm and an absolute displacement of more than 10 mm on the affected knee have a sensitivity of 99% for a torn ACL.[4] We have used the KT-1000 extensively since the mid-1980s and have found that patients are very receptive to its use. In fact, many are very pleased to have an objective measure to confirm the absence or integrity of the anterior cruciate ligament.

Plain radiographs are typically normal in an acute ACL injury. However, plain radiographs should always be obtained to rule out associated fractures. The Segond fracture, a lateral capsular avulsion, is very closely correlated with ACL injury.[5] It is noted just distal to the tibial articular surface on the anterior aspect of the tibia. Tibial eminence fractures are infrequent but can be seen in adolescents or in those patients with diminished bone mineral density (Figures 2-2A to 2-2C). Furthermore, in adolescent patients, one can assess the physis to determine skeletal maturity, though we generally use the more standardized posterior–anterior (PA) left-hand bone age to assess skeletal age.[6]

In chronic ACL-deficient knees, periarticular spurring may be noted. The tunnel view (PA flexed knee view) may show intercondylar notch osteophytes and blunting of the tibial eminences. A depression in the lateral femoral condyle was initially noted in chronically ACL-deficient knees.[7] This lateral notch sign occurs when the normal sulcus terminalis on the lateral femoral condyle becomes more prominent and has been associated with chronic ACL deficiency.[8] Other reports have noted this sign even in acute tears, especially in younger males with concomitant lateral meniscal tears.[9]

MRI is helpful in assessing bone contusions (bone bruises), tibial eminence fractures, intra-articular fractures, associated collateral ligament injuries, as well as articular cartilage and meniscal pathologies. MRI evaluation of the knee requires images in the coronal, sagittal, and axial planes. Imaging sequences include T2-weighted with fast spin echo and fat saturation or short tau inversion recovery (STIR) performed in all three planes to

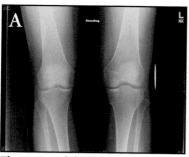
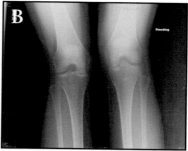
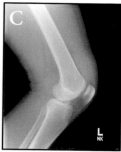

Figure 2-2. (A) AP (anterior to posterior) standing radiographs demonstrating a nondisplaced tibial spine fracture of the left knee. (B) PA (posterior to anterior) flexed knee standing radiograph demonstrating the tibial spine fracture on the left knee. (C) Lateral radiograph demonstrating the tibial spine fracture.

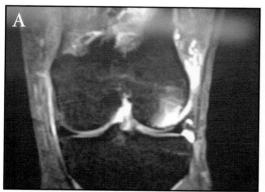
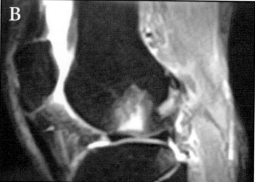

Figure 2-3. (A) Coronal and (B) sagittal MRIs demonstrating lateral compartment bone bruise.

assess pathology including the muscles, tendons, ligaments, and articular cartilage. These sequences also accurately depict edema and bone bruises. T1 and proton density sequences highlight anatomy and should be performed in the sagittal and coronal planes. These are most accurate in diagnosing meniscal tears.[10] Sanders and Miller outlined direct and indirect signs of ACL disruption found on MRI.[10]

* Direct signs
   * Discontinuity of fibers
   * Abnormal slope of ACL
   * Nonvisualization on both sagital and coronal planes
   * Avulsion fracture of the tibial spine
* Indirect signs
   * Bone contusion sign: lateral femoral condyle and posterior tibial plateau (Figures 2-3A and 2-3B)
   * Deep sulcus sign: lateral femoral condyle (more than 2 mm deep)
   * Segond fracture: capsular avulsion fracture of the lateral tibial plateau
   * Kissing contusions: anterior tibia and femur (hyperextension injury)
   * Anterior drawer sign: anterior translation of tibia relative to femur

❖ Buckling of PCL: nonspecific

❖ Acute hemarthrosis: nonspecific

The bone bruise is typically seen only in acutely injured knees and rarely found in chronically ACL-deficient knees. It is found in the lateral compartment, in the middle third of the lateral femoral condyle and in the posterior third of the lateral tibial plateau in the sagittal plane.[11]

While MRI is tremendously useful in the ACL-injured kneed, it does not replace careful physical exam, as studies have demonstrated that physical exam by a skilled practitioner is at least as accurate as MRI in the diagnosis of meniscal and ACL pathology. Furthermore, MRI is not useful in differentiating partial and complete ACL tears.[12]

In summary, a careful physical exam is the most important test in the assessment of an injured knee. The KT-1000 arthrometer is an especially useful adjunct to the physical exam, and when one finds translation values of greater than 10 mm on maximum manual testing, a side-to-side difference of greater than 3 mm, and a compliance index of 2 mm or more, the examiner can be certain of ACL deficiency. Plain x-rays assist the physician in ruling out associated fractures and in assessing the overall morphology of the articular surfaces of the joint. MRI scanning reveals bone bruises and meniscal and collateral ligament injuries and can help confirm the diagnosis of ACL injury in the setting of equivocal physical exam and KT-1000 measurements.

References

1. Fetto J, Marshall J. Injury to the anterior cruciate ligament producing the pivot-shift sign. *J Bone Joint Surg.* 1979;61-A:710-714.
2. Daniel D, Stone M, Sachs R, Malcolm L. Instrumented measurement of anterior knee laxity in patients with acute anterior cruciate ligament disruption. *Am J Sports Med.* 1985;13:401-407.
3. Bach BJ, Warren R, Flynn W, Kroll M, Wickiewiecz T. Arthrometric evaluation of knees that have a torn anterior cruciate ligament. *J Bone Joint Surg.* 1990;72-A:1299-1306.
4. Alford J, Bach BJ. Arthrometric aspects of anterior cruciate ligament surgery before and after reconstruction with patellar tendon grafts. *Tech Orthop.* 2005;20:421-438.
5. Hess T, Rupp S, Hopf T, Gleitz M, Liebler J. Lateral tibial avulsion fractures and disruptions to the anterior cruciate ligament. *Clin Orthop.* 1994;303:193-197.
6. Greulich W, Pyle S. *Radiographic Atlas of Skeletal Development of the Hand and Wrist.* Stanford, CA: Stanford University Press; 1959.
7. Losee R, Johnson T, Southwick W. Anterior subluxation of the lateral tibial plateau. A diagnostic test and operative repair. *J Bone Joint Surg.* 1978;60-A:1015-1030.
8. Warren R, Kaplan N, Bach BJ. The lateral notch sign of anterior cruciate ligament insufficiency. *Am J Knee Surg.* 1988;1:119-124.
9. Garth W, Greco J, House M. The lateral notch sign associated with acute anterior cruciate ligament disruption. *Am J Sports Med.* 2000;28:68-73.
10. Sanders T, Miller M. A systematic approach to magnetic resonance imaging interpretation of sports medicine injuries of the knee. *Am J Sports Med.* 2005;33:131-148.
11. Graf B, Cook D, DeSmet A, Kleene J. "Bone bruises" on magnetic resonance imaging evaluation of anterior cruciate ligament injuries. *Am J Sports Med.* 1993;21:220-223.
12. Bach BJ, Nho S. Anterior cruciate ligament: diagnosis and decision making. In: Miller M, Cole B, eds. *Textbook of Arthroscopy.* Philadelphia, PA: Saunders; 2004:633-643.

HOW DO YOU MANAGE A COMBINED ACL/MCL INJURY?

Anne E. Colton, MD, and Charles A. Bush-Joseph, MD

The anterior cruciate ligament (ACL) prevents anterior translation of the tibia on the femur and contributes to resistance to internal and external rotation while the knee is extended. It is a secondary stabilizer to valgus stress in full extension. The medial collateral ligament (MCL) resists valgus stress at 30 degrees of knee flexion. It also contributes to limiting anterior and posterior translation, as well as rotation, of the tibia. Thus, when both ligaments are disrupted, the knee can become unstable in several planes of function.

MCL injuries are classified as grade I, II, or III, as described by the American Medical Association's *Ligament Injury Classification*.[1] A grade I injury indicates a microscopic tearing of the ligament without laxity. A grade II is a partial tear of the ligament with some joint widening but not a complete disruption. On physical examination, there remains a firm endpoint on valgus (abduction) testing. A grade III injury implies loss of integrity of the ligament, with medial joint widening and a soft or nonexistent endpoint upon valgus (abduction) stress.

ACL rupture along with MCL rupture can seriously compromise joint stability.[2] These injuries can be difficult to treat. Multiple studies have shown that concomitant ACL reconstruction and MCL repair can lead to postoperative arthrofibrosis. However, persistent valgus instability in cases when the MCL is not repaired can compromise the results of the ACL reconstruction. Thus, I have developed this algorithm:

* When a patient has a grade I MCL injury with concomitant ACL disruption, I treat this as an isolated ACL and reconstruct the ACL as soon as full range of motion is achieved.

* In grade II MCL injuries, I treat the patient in a hinged knee brace for 3 to 6 weeks, achieve full range of motion, and reconstruct the ACL when motion returns and valgus stability is established.

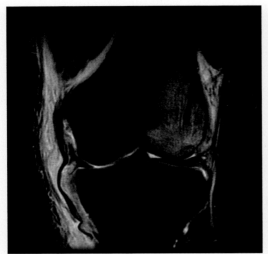

Figure 3-1. T2-weighted coronal MRI shows the distal avulsion of the MCL.

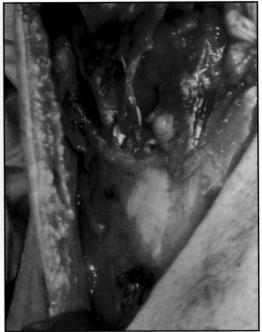

Figure 3-2. Intraoperative photograph showing the distal MCL avulsion repaired over a staple post.

＊ A grade III MCL injury implies a complete rupture of the superficial and deep ligament, resulting in incompetence of the medial knee structures. Magnetic resonance imaging (MRI) can detect the exact location of the tear of the MCL.[3] For a distal avulsion (off the tibia), which is superficial ligament disruption along with deep meniscotibial ligament failure (Figure 3-1), I opt for acute fixation of the MCL with concomitant reconstruction of the ACL. I believe that persistent synovial fluid under the ligament from disruption of the medial capsule prevents adequate healing of the ligament to bone.

For this distal avulsion of the MCL, I utilize suture anchors for the deeper fibers of the MCL if the meniscus is subluxated and most often secure the distal aspect of the ligament (the superficial ligament) over a staple post (Figure 3-2), passing under the pes tendons, with the knee in extension. I take care to ensure that this repair is done at the isometric point, as overtightening the ligament can result in motion restriction. Figures 3-3 and 3-4 show postoperative radiographs following ACL reconstruction with MCL repair. Fixation can also be accomplished with a screw and soft tissue washer.

Postoperatively, I treat the patients with combined ACL and MCL injuries with reconstruction/repair in a hinged knee brace for approximately 3 to 4 weeks. Range of motion exercises and quadriceps strengthening exercises are begun 1 to 2 days following surgery.

A prospective randomized study by Halinen et al[4] compared 2 groups of patients with combined ACL and grade III MCL ruptures. One group had ACL reconstruction alone; the other group had concomitant MCL repair. There was no significant difference

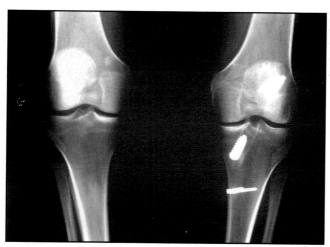

Figure 3-3. Postoperative anteroposterior (AP) x-ray after ACL reconstruction with bone-patellar tendon-bone (BTB) autograft and MCL repair over a staple.

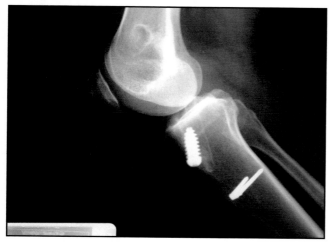

Figure 3-4. Postoperative lateral x-ray showing the fixation of both the ACL and MCL grafts.

in outcomes between the 2 groups at an average follow-up of 27 months. Shelbourne and Porter[5] compared groups of patients with these combined ligament injuries who either underwent ACL reconstruction alone or who underwent ACL reconstruction with MCL repair. The authors found that these 2 groups had no difference in valgus laxity, range of motion, or subjective measures.

Hillard-Sembell and her coauthors[6] found no late instability among 3 different groups of patients: ACL reconstruction and MCL repair, ACL reconstruction only, and nonoperative treatment for both. They retrospectively reviewed 66 patients at an average follow-up of 45 months. While there was no clinical instability evident, there was increased medial side opening on stress radiographs in 8 patients, 6 of whom had not undergone an MCL repair. Because of the small numbers, however, there was no significance found in this outcome.

Nakamura's MRI study[3] concluded that the location of the MCL injury can predict the outcome of nonsurgical treatment of MCL injuries in combination with ACL reconstruction. Eleven of 17 patients had regained valgus stability at 6 weeks after bracing, and they underwent lone ACL reconstruction. All but one of these patients had an MCL lesion at the femoral attachment site. Six patients whose injury was extensile from the femoral epicondyle to the joint line had residual instability and went on to have surgical intervention for both the ACL and MCL. These findings are consistent with what I have seen in my practice.

References

1. American Medical Association. *Standard Nomenclature of Athletic Injuries*. Chicago, IL: American Medical Association; 1966:99-100.
2. Noyes FR, Barber-Westin SD. The treatment of acute combined ruptures of the anterior cruciate and medial ligaments of the knee. *Am J Sports Med*. 1995;23:380-389.
3. Nakamura N, Horibe S, Toritsuka Y, Mitsuoka T, Yoshikawa H, Shino K. Acute grade III medial collateral ligament injury of the knee associated with anterior cruciate ligament tear. The usefulness of magnetic resonance imaging in determining a treatment regimen. *Am J Sports Med*. 2003;31:261-267.
4. Halinen J, Lindahl J, Hirvensalo E, Santavirta S. Operative and nonoperative treatments of medial collateral ligament rupture with early anterior cruciate ligament reconstruction: a prospective randomized study. *Am J Sports Med*. 2006;34:1134-1140.
5. Shelbourne, KD, Porter DA. Anterior cruciate ligament-medial collateral ligament injury: Nonoperative management of medial collateral ligament tears with anterior cruciate ligament reconstruction. A preliminary report. *Am J Sports Med*. 1992;20:283-286.
6. Hillard-Sembell D, Daniel DM, Stone ML, Dobson BE, Fithian DC. Combined injuries of the anterior cruciate and medial collateral ligaments of the knee. Effect of treatment on stability and function of the joint. *J Bone Joint Surg Am*. 1996;78:169-176.

How Do You Manage a Combined ACL/LCL Injury?

Anne E. Colton, MD, and Charles A. Bush-Joseph, MD

The lateral collateral ligament (LCL) is the primary static restraint to varus stress of the knee at 30 degrees of knee flexion. It also contributes to resistance to external rotation and anterior translation of the tibia on the femur. More typically, the LCL is injured along with the other posterolateral structures of the knee. Injury to the LCL along with the anterior cruciate ligament (ACL) can dramatically increase varus and external rotation instability, and a missed LCL or other posterolateral corner injury is a major cause for failure of ACL reconstruction.[1]

In an ACL rupture, the radiographic sign of a Segond fracture indicates a lateral capsule avulsion. It is not, however, an indicator of injury to the posterolateral corner. In an LCL/posterolateral corner of injury one may see an avulsion of the fibular styloid or the lateral femoral epicondyle with LCL injuries or a Gerdy's tubercle avulsion with an iliotibial band injury.

I treat these injuries as acutely as possible, as soon as range of motion is maximized and swelling has decreased. This is typically within 2 weeks of injury. Early reconstruction is imperative, as delayed diagnosis and repair can lead to scar formation, distortion of soft tissue planes, and difficulty in identifying injured structures for repair. If necessary, the procedure can be staged to complete the open lateral repair early, with a staged endoscopic ACL reconstruction at a later date. I no longer utilize primary repair alone, and in almost all cases I augment the repair with allograft tissue.

For an LCL injury, I utilize the docking technique, first described by Rohrburg[2] in the elbow for medial collateral ligament (MCL) reconstruction and then adapted to the posterolateral corner by Verma.[3] I first reconstruct the ACL endoscopically. After this has been accomplished, I make a separate lateral incision for the LCL repair. Utilizing this approach, extending from the lateral epicondyle to the anterior aspect of the fibula, I take the incision down to the iliotibial band, raising skin flaps. The peroneal nerve posterior

Figure 4-1. Semitendinosis allograft passed through fibular tunnel and passed under the iliotibial band.

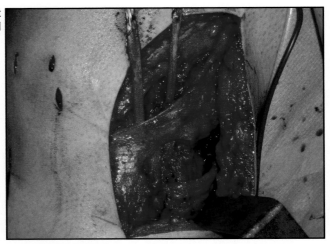

Figure 4-2. Each limb of the graft is docked into the femoral epicondyle tunnel.

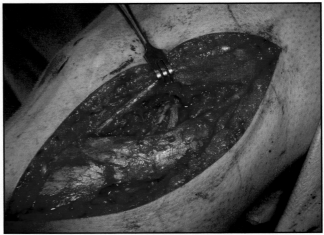

to the biceps femoris is isolated and protected throughout the procedure. The iliotibial band is incised longitudinally along its fibers, and the disrupted LCL is exposed. The fibular head is exposed subperiostally. If this is a distal avulsion injury, I typically reattach it through drill holes through the fibular head, taking care to protect the peroneal nerve. A midsubstance tear can be repaired primarily using Bunnell-type suturing. If this is a proximal avulsion, I often use suture anchors or transosseous drill holes to reapproximate the LCL to the lateral epicondyle. The repair is most commonly augmented with an allograft semitendinosis reconstruction. The tunnel (usually 6 to 8 mm) is drilled anterior to posterior through the fibula. The graft is threaded through this tunnel and passed under the iliotibial band (Figure 4-1). A drill hole is made anterior to the lateral femoral epicondyle at the isometric point. Each limb of the graft is then passed through the tunnel and given appropriate tension, with the knee flexed slightly and gentle valgus stress applied (Figure 4-2). An interference screw is then placed to complete this docking technique.

Complications of this surgery include overconstraint of the knee from overtightening of the ligaments, arthrofibrosis, and hardware complications.

Latimer et al[4] reported on 10 patients with combined cruciate and posterolateral instability who were reconstructed with a bone-patellar tendon-bone (BTB) allograft fixed with interference screws in tunnels place in the fibular head and the isometric point at the lateral femoral epicondyle. Six out of the 10 patients had no varus laxity, and 4 had 1+ laxity at an average follow-up of 28 months. Nine out of 10 had resumed full range of motion.

References

1. O'Brien SJ, Warren RF, Pavlov H, Panariello R, Wickiewicz TL. Reconstruction of the chronically insufficient anterior cruciate ligament with the central third of the patellar ligament. *J Bone Joint Surg Am.* 1991;73(2):278-286.
2. Rohrbough, JT, Altcheck DW, Hyman J, Williams RJ III, Botts JD. Medical collateral ligament reconstruction of the elbow using the docking technique. *Am J Sports Med.* 2002;30:540-548.
3. Verma NN, Mithofer K, Battaglia M, MacGillivray J. The docking technique for posterolateral corner reconstruction. *Arthroscopy.* 2005;21:238-242.
4. Latimer HA, Tibone JE, ElAttrache NS, McMahon PJ. Reconstruction of the lateral collateral ligament with patellar tendon allograft: report of a new technique in combined ligament injuries. *Am J Sports Med.* 1998;26: 656-662.

WHAT DETERMINES WHICH GRAFT YOU RECOMMEND FOR ACL SURGERY?

Anne E. Colton, MD, and Charles A. Bush-Joseph, MD

There are many factors to consider when choosing a graft for anterior cruciate ligament reconstruction. The patient's activity level, age, comorbidities, and ability to rehabilitate all contribute to the decision among the differing types of anterior cruciate ligament (ACL) grafts for reconstruction. The choice of graft varies in biologic aspect of healing, biomechanical properties, graft harvest morbidity, fixation options, and return-to-play and rehabilitation guidelines. Graft choices include bone-patellar tendon-bone (BTB), quadrupled hamstring tendon autograft (QHA), quadriceps tendon, Achilles, posterior tibialis, fascia lata, and tibialis anterior allografts. The most commonly used grafts are the BTB and QHA.

The native ACL has an ultimate tensile load of 2160 N and a stiffness of 242 N/mm.[1] The BTB graft has an ultimate tensile load of 2977 N and a stiffness of 620 N/mm,[1,2] whereas the QHA, comprised of the semitendinosis and gracilis tendons, has an ultimate tensile load of 4090 N and a stiffness of 776 N/mm.[3] Ideally, I would like a graft that most closely approximates the native ACL, although graft biomechanical properties are reduced following surgical reconstruction. Thus, I also rely on other factors to make my ultimate decision regarding graft choice.

Typically in an active patient population under the age of 30 with a primary ACL rupture, I recommend autograft ACL reconstruction. This eliminates the risk (albeit low) of virus or other disease transmission in allograft transplantation. The 2 potential autograft harvests I utilize are quadrupled hamstrings (QHA, Figure 5-1) and BTB. For the highly competitive athletes, such as those on the collegiate and professional level, as well as high school athletes with a desire to play competitively in college, I usually use a BTB. The biologic advantage of bone-to-bone healing (similar to fracture healing) enables earlier incorporation of the graft, leading to quicker return to play. These can be rehabilitated at a faster pace. Studies have shown that graft incorporation occurs within 6 weeks'

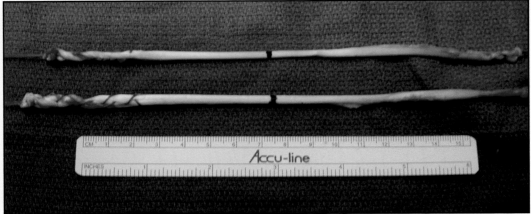

Figure 5-1. Semitendinosis and gracilis tendons for quadrupled hamstring autograft ACL reconstruction.

Figure 5-2. Bone-patellar-bone allograft.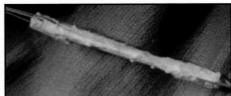

time, as opposed to 8 to 12 weeks in a hamstring autograft.[4] In addition, they do not have the hamstring weakness that can occur from harvesting the hamstring autograft. Quadrupled hamstrings, however, are stronger and stiffer than the other choices[3,4] and do not have the donor site morbidity (ie, the anterior knee pain, problems with kneeling, etc). Lower demand athletes can have excellent results with the QHA.

I recommend allograft BTB (Figure 5-2) in patients who wish minimum surgical morbidity, those with significant arthrosis, and older patients. For patients who have a questionable ability to rehabilitate, for reasons of obesity or lack of compliance or motivation, I feel that an allograft is the best choice. In addition, there is a subset of patients who have a history of patellofemoral pain or patellofemoral malalignment that may put them at risk for worsened outcomes following BTB autograft harvest. With allograft BTB, there is no donor site morbidity, abundant availability of larger graft sources, and better cosmesis with smaller scars. However, with a donor tendon, concerns remain about the disease transmission, slower graft incorporation, increased immunologic-mediated inflammatory response, and persistent effusion. It is important to counsel patients adequately regarding these risks.

References

1. Woo SL-Y, Hollis JM, Adams DJ, Lyon RM, Takai S. Tensile properties of the human femur-anterior cruciate ligament-tibia complex. *Am J Sports Med.* 1991;19:217-225.
2. Noyes FR, Butler DL, Grood ES, Zernicke RF, Hefzy MS. Biomechanical analysis of human ligament grafts used in knee-ligament repairs and reconstructions. *J Bone J Surg Am.* 1984;66:344-352.

3. Hamner DL, Brown CH Jr, Steiner ME, Hecker AT, Hayes WC. Hamstring tendon grafts for reconstruction of the anterior cruciate ligament: biomechanical evaluation of the use of multiple strands and tensioning techniques. *J Bone Joint Surg Am.* 1999;81:549-557.
4. Rodeo SA, Arnoczky SP, Torzilli PA, Hidaka C, Warren RF. Tendon-healing in a bone tunnel: a biomechanical and histological study in the dog. *J Bone Joint Surg Am.* 1993;75:1795-1803.

WHEN WOULD YOU USE PATELLAR TENDON AUTOGRAFT AS YOUR MAIN GRAFT SELECTION?

John-Paul H. Rue, MD, LCDR, MC, USN, and Brian J. Cole, MD, MBA

I use patellar tendon autograft as my main graft selection in young, high-demand, active patients. Bone-patellar tendon-bone (BTB) autograft anterior cruciate ligament (ACL) reconstruction has the longest proven record of successful outcomes and is the technique by which all others are compared (Table 6-1). We believe that this graft may also have some advantages for a subset of high-demand patients who desire or require a quick return to cutting and pivoting sports. Specifically, BTB autograft allows for bone-to-bone fixation with metal interference screws, which has been shown to be a strong and reliable fixation method with an initial fixation strength of 558 Newtons (N).[5] Additionally, there is evidence to support using BTB autograft in order to minimize hamstring avoidance, especially in young female soccer players.[6] For these several reasons, BTB autograft is our graft of choice for young, high-demand, active patients without preexisting anterior knee pain (Figure 6-1).

I would not use patellar tendon autograft in patients with preexisting anterior knee pain or in those patients who do a large amount of kneeling for work or religion because they may be more likely to have anterior knee pain from the graft harvest site[7] (Figure 6-1). This is controversial because it has been shown that there is no difference in the incidence of anterior knee pain between patients with bone-patellar tendon-bone autografts and allografts.[8] There is, however, probably a trend toward more anterior knee pain with patellar tendon autograft ACL reconstructions when compared to hamstring autograft ACL reconstructions.[9]

Deciding which graft to recommend to a patient for ACL reconstruction involves many factors. Ideally, an ACL graft should have biomechanical and structural properties that are similar to those of the patient's own ACL. The initial graft tensile strength of bone-patellar tendon-bone autograft is 2977 N with a stiffness of 620 N/mm. This is over 1.5 times the strength and 4 times the stiffness of the native ACL.[10,11] Additionally, graft

Table 6-1

Bone-Patellar Tendon-Bone Anterior Cruciate Ligament Reconstruction Outcomes

Author and Year Published	# Patients	Average Follow-up (Months)	KT-1000 Arthrometer Side-to-Side Difference < 3 mm (% of Patients)	Pivot Shift Grade 0 (% of Patients)	Post-operative Knee Scores
Patel et al 2000[1]	32	70	88	91	Lysholm (mean) 89
Corry et al 1999[2]	82	24	91	91	IKDC* 80%
Bach et al 1998[3]	97	79	70	84	Lysholm (mean) 87
Webb et al 1998[4]	82	24	90	91	Lysholm (mean) 93 IKDC 86%

*IKDC = International Knee Documentation Committee.

Figure 6-1. Skin markings for BTB auto-graft harvest.

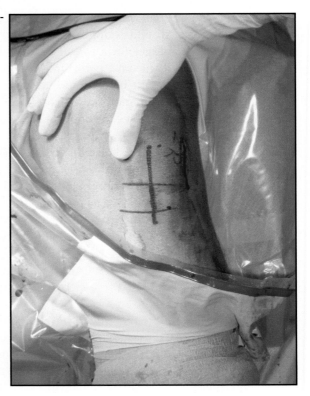

fixation should be secure enough to allow early rehabilitation with rapid incorporation of the graft. Bone-patellar tendon-bone autograft allows for bone-to-bone healing with metal interference screws, one of the most secure methods of fixation.

I believe that the choice of which graft to use should come from a thorough discussion of the risks and benefits of all available choices and should ultimately be an informed decision by the patient. In a systematic review of 9 randomized controlled studies comparing patellar tendon and hamstring tendon autografts, Spindler et al found no significant difference in failure rates between graft sources.[12] This suggests that there may be no significant difference in outcomes among properly performed ACL reconstructions with different graft sources. Certainly, a surgeon's comfort level with a particular graft selection should play a role in deciding which graft a patient chooses. Regardless of graft choice, the best chance for a successful outcome will come from a well-planned and properly performed surgery. For most surgeons, this will be accomplished by performing the technique that he or she is most familiar with and comfortable performing.

Disclaimer

The views expressed in this article are those of the author and do not necessarily reflect the official policy or position of the Department of the Navy, Department of Defense, nor the United States Government.

References

1. Patel D, Church J, Hall A. Central third bone-patellar tendon-bone anterior cruciate ligament reconstruction: a 5-year follow-up. *Arthroscopy.* 2000;16:67-70.
2. Corry I, Webb J, Clingeleffer A, Pinczewski L. Arthroscopic reconstruction of the anterior cruciate ligament. A comparison of patellar tendon autograft and four-strand hamstring tendon autograft. *Am J Sports Med.* 1999; 27:444-454.
3. Bach B, Tradonsky S, Bojchuk J, Levy M, Bush-Joseph C, Khan N. Arthroscopically assisted anterior cruciate ligament reconstruction using patellar tendon autograft. Five- to nine-year follow-up evaluation. *Am J Sports Med.* 1998;26:20-29.
4. Webb J, Corry I, Clingeleffer A, Pinczewski L. Endoscopic reconstruction for isolated anterior cruciate ligament rupture. *J Bone Joint Surg Br.* 1998;80:288-294.
5. Jackson D, Grood E, Goldstein J, et al. A comparison of patellar tendon autograft and allograft used for anterior cruciate ligament reconstruction in the goat model. *Am J Sports Med.* 1993;21:176-185.
6. Hewett T, Myer G, Ford K. Anterior cruciate ligament injuries in female athletes: part 1, mechanisms and risk factors. *Am J Sports Med.* 2006;34.
7. Phelan D, Cohen A, Fithian D. Complications of anterior cruciate ligament reconstruction. *Instr Course Lect.* 2006;55:465-474.
8. Shelton W, Papendick L, Dukes A. Autograft versus allograft anterior cruciate ligament reconstruction. *Arthroscopy.* 1997;13(4):446-449.
9. Freedman K, D'Amato M, Nedeff D, Kaz A, Bach BJ. Arthroscopic anterior cruciate ligament reconstruction: a metaanalysis comparing patellar tendon and hamstring tendon autografts. *Am J Knee Surg.* 2003;31:2-11.
10. West R, Harner C. Graft selection in anterior cruciate ligament reconstruction. *J Am Acad Orthop Surg.* 2005;13:197-207.
11. Noyes F, Butler D, Grood E, Zernicke R, Hefzy M. Biomechanical analysis of human ligament grafts used in knee-ligament repairs and reconstructions. *J Bone Joint Surg Am.* 1984;66:344-352.
12. Spindler K, Kuhn J, Freedman K, Matthews C, Dittus R, Harrell F. Anterior cruciate ligament reconstruction autograft choice: bone-tendon-bone versus hamstring. Does it really matter? A systematic review. *Am J Sports Med.* 2004;32:1986-1995.

WHEN WOULD YOU USE HAMSTRING AUTOGRAFT AS YOUR MAIN GRAFT SOURCE?

Matthew T. Provencher, MD, LCDR, MC, USN, and Nikhil N. Verma, MD

A continuing debate remains regarding the optimal graft for anterior cruciate ligament (ACL) reconstruction. While the bone-tendon-bone autograft has traditionally been regarded as the gold standard for ACL surgery, there is continued interest in the use of soft tissue autografts, which include the hamstring tendons (semitendinosus and gracilis). The ideal ACL reconstruction graft retains biomechanical properties similar to the native ligament, possesses vascular channels and healing potential, and behaves as a ligament, with appropriate collagen cross-linking and parallel nature of the collagen fibrils. With an estimated ultimate strength of 2150 N (Newtons) and stiffness of 240 N/mm,[1] the biomechanics of the native ACL can be met or surpassed by many available autograft constructs. Multiple studies have demonstrated that the doubled semitendinosus/gracilis (hamstring [HS]) autograft has superior strength (4500 N) and stiffness (800 N/mm) to a bone-patellar tendon-bone (BTB) autograft (2900 N strength, 455 N/mm).[2,3] Thus, each graft construct meets or exceeds the native ligament; however, it is well known that fixation, especially on the tibial side, is the weak link of the construct. With the recent improvement in fixation techniques for soft-tissue tendons, the concern for soft-tissue healing problems is becoming less. Additionally, several randomized studies have supported the use of both graft constructs, especially in terms of patient satisfaction, activity level, and knee function.[4-12]

When determining which autograft to offer a patient, one should keep in mind several additional factors that may alter the performance of the knee after autograft harvest. Each autograft (BTB or HS) has inherent donor site morbidity issues that need to be recognized and discussed with the patient. Although not all surgeons perform both types of reconstructive procedures and usually have more experience with one technique over the other, some have recommended a patient-customized approach to graft selection after a relative discussion of the risks and benefits of each. There are also certain situations when you would want to clearly recommend one graft over the other to your patient (see Table 7-1).

Table 7-1

Indications for Hamstring Versus Bone-Patellar-Bone Autograft

Diagnosis	Patient History	Physical Examination or Radiographic Findings
Strong Indications for HS Autograft Over BTB Autograft		
Patellar tendonitis	Jumper's knee, anterior knee pain	Tenderness at distal pole of patella or in tendon, esp. with resisted flexion
Active or chronic patellar instability, subluxation, or dislocation history	Patellar subluxation or dislocation, possibly reduced on the field or in the ER	Patellar apprehension, positive J-sign, increased patellar instability laterally
Chondral damage to the patellofemoral joint, may not be symptomatic	Pain with flexion and extension of the knee in the trochlear area, possibly audible crepitus	Crepitus in the patellofemoral joint, compression pain
Patella infera	Congenital or acquired through prior patellar injury	Insufficient graft length as evidence on the lateral 45 degrees radiograph
Bipartite patella, with a large component	Either symptomatic or asymptomatic patellar pain	Tenderness in the superolateral patella, worse with resisted flexion
Lesser Indications for HS Autograft Over BTB Autograft		
Prior patellar tendon repair or rupture	Patient history	Surgical scars present
Occupational or vocation activities in the prone position	Roofers, tile layers, flooring work, plumbers, and certain military personnel	May have multiple abrasions or old scars over the patella
Sporting requirements; may be contraindication to HS autograft	Sprinters, high jumpers, hurdlers require high peak flexion torque, which may be decreased after HS harvest	May not offer HS in these sports
Donor site morbidity	Numbness in the anterior knee	Document intact infrapatellar branch of the saphenous nerve
S/P prior BTB harvest, revision ACL reconstruction required	Patient had prior BTB primary reconstruction	May be concern for reharvest if MRI shows thinning or gap formation in the tendon

There are several preexisting conditions for which an HS autograft should be considered as the primary graft source over BTB. These factors can be broken down into patellofemoral disorders, revision surgery after a primary BTB surgery, occupational issues, and athletic concerns.

The patellofemoral joint in any patient undergoing an ACL reconstruction deserves careful scrutiny. First, the patient should be questioned regarding the presence or absence of anterior knee pain, jumper's knee, patellar tendonitis history, prior patellar injury, subluxation, or dislocation that has occurred with either occupational or vocational activities. The physical examination of the patellofemoral joint should focus on symptomatic patellar crepitus, compression pain, patellar instability, and patellar mobility. The radiographs, especially the 45 degrees lateral and direct anteroposterior (AP) view, should be obtained to assess for prior malunion or nonunion after patellar fracture, the presence of a bipartite patellar (especially in the superolateral aspect), and concern for patellar infera (insufficient graft material) or alta. Any patient with a symptomatic patellofemoral joint, or radiographic abnormalities to suggest that the BTB harvest may be compromised, should be offered a HS graft as a primary construct.[4,13]

Anterior knee pain is a phenomenon well known after BTB reconstruction;[4,6,8-13] however, the HS autograft is not without evidence of postoperative anterior knee pain. Regardless, most studies have suggested that the anterior knee pain that may occur after BTB ACL reconstruction may be profound and limits patients in certain occupational or sporting activities. All patients should be questioned as to their occupation and sporting/vocational activities. If there is an indication that the patient may spend a large amount of time in the prone position (roofing industry, tile, flooring, plumbing, etc), or those in the military who are often in the prone position (riflemen, ground troops), an HS autograft should be considered.[4,6,13] The presence of anterior knee pain after HS reconstruction has been consistently shown to be less than BTB, although it is still present. The occupational status for graft choice is a relative indication for HS autograft, and it deserves discussion with your patient.

Certain sporting activities may make a patient prone to dysfunction after autograft HS reconstruction. It has been demonstrated that the peak flexion torque at high amounts of knee flexion is reduced after autograft HS harvest.[14,15] This may make it difficult for athletes who require high-flexion torque, such as high jumpers, long jumpers, and hurdlers. Interestingly, patients who wear cowboy boots often complain of slight weakness or knee pain in the HS harvest region while taking their boots off, which requires a high-flexion position and some level of knee flexion torque. However, the BTB reconstruction is not without some level of dysfunction in the quadriceps. This is debatable and may be due solely to the surgery of ACL reconstruction itself and not due to patellar tendon harvest, as both quadriceps and HS power loss (up to 10%) were noted in a prospective comparison of both HS and BTB graft groups.[13] Others[16] have found no difference at 2-year follow-up with regards to peak torque in extension and flexion after both graft types, whereas hamstring power loss up to 50% after HS grafting, most notably in flexion torque beyond 60 degrees of flexion, and 50% quadriceps extension loss after BTB graft have been documented.[17] Strength and knee positional torque loss after either autograft remains debatable; however, one should discuss the potential losses that are usually associated with each graft type.

Donor site morbidity is a concern after harvest of either autograft. The BTB harvest may have a higher rate of injury to the infrapatellar branch of the saphenous nerve, but this has also been described in HS harvest. The HS harvest can usually be accomplished through a smaller incision with potentially less donor site morbidity.[13] Painful scars have been described after BTB harvest that may be especially sensitive while doing prone position work with an anterior load on the patella. However, pes anserine bursitis may develop after HS harvest and can be particularly debilitating to recovery and overall knee function.[13]

Finally, preoperative advanced imaging studies (magnetic resonance imaging [MRI]) may offer some relative guidance to harvest the HS autograft primarily. Patients who are identified as having a large and near-full-thickness chondral injury in the trochlea or patella, even if asymptomatic, may be made symptomatic by BTB autograft harvest, as it has been shown that patellofemoral contact pressures may be increased after patellar bone block harvest.[18] However, it is not known whether the HS may cause an identical problem.

References

1. Woo SL, Hollis JM, Adams DJ, Lyon RM, Takai S. Tensile properties of the human femur-anterior cruciate ligament-tibia complex. The effects of specimen age and orientation. *Am J Sports Med*. 1991;19(3):217-225.
2. Cooper DE, Deng XH, Burstein AL, Warren RF. The strength of the central third patellar tendon graft. A biomechanical study. *Am J Sports Med*. 1993;21(6):818-823; discussion 823-814.
3. Hamner DL, Brown CH Jr, Steiner ME, Hecker AT, Hayes WC. Hamstring tendon grafts for reconstruction of the anterior cruciate ligament: biomechanical evaluation of the use of multiple strands and tensioning techniques. *J Bone Joint Surg Am*. 1999;81(4):549-557.
4. Aune AK, Holm I, Risberg MA, Jensen HK, Steen H. Four-strand hamstring tendon autograft compared with patellar tendon-bone autograft for anterior cruciate ligament reconstruction. A randomized study with two-year follow-up. *Am J Sports Med*. 2001;29(6):722-728.
5. Ejerhed L, Kartus J, Sernert N, Kohler K, Karlsson J. Patellar tendon or semitendinosus tendon autografts for anterior cruciate ligament reconstruction? A prospective randomized study with a two-year follow-up. *Am J Sports Med*. 2003;31(1):19-25.
6. Freedman KB, D'Amato MJ, Nedeff DD, Kaz A, Bach BR Jr. Arthroscopic anterior cruciate ligament reconstruction: a metaanalysis comparing patellar tendon and hamstring tendon autografts. *Am J Sports Med*. 2003; 31(1):2-11.
7. Jansson KA, Linko E, Sandelin J, Harilainen A. A prospective randomized study of patellar versus hamstring tendon autografts for anterior cruciate ligament reconstruction. *Am J Sports Med*. 2003;31(1):12-18.
8. Laxdal G, Sernert N, Ejerhed L, Karlsson J, Kartus JT. A prospective comparison of bone-patellar tendon-bone and hamstring tendon grafts for anterior cruciate ligament reconstruction in male patients. *Knee Surg Sports Traumatol Arthrosc*. 2007;15(2):113-114.
9. Roe J, Pinczewski LA, Russell VJ, Salmon LJ, Kawamata T, Chew M. A 7-year follow-up of patellar tendon and hamstring tendon grafts for arthroscopic anterior cruciate ligament reconstruction: differences and similarities. *Am J Sports Med*. 2005;33(9):1337-1345.
10. Sajovic M, Vengust V, Komadina R, Tavcar R, Skaza K. A prospective, randomized comparison of semitendinosus and gracilis tendon versus patellar tendon autografts for anterior cruciate ligament reconstruction: five-year follow-up. *Am J Sports Med*. 2006;34(12):1933-1940.
11. Shaieb MD, Kan DM, Chang SK, Marumoto JM, Richardson AB. A prospective randomized comparison of patellar tendon versus semitendinosus and gracilis tendon autografts for anterior cruciate ligament reconstruction. *Am J Sports Med*. 2002;30(2):214-220.
12. Spindler KP, Kuhn JE, Freedman KB, Matthews CE, Dittus RS, Harrell FE Jr. Anterior cruciate ligament reconstruction autograft choice: bone-tendon-bone versus hamstring: does it really matter? A systematic review. *Am J Sports Med*. 2004;32(8):1986-1995.
13. Bartlett RJ, Clatworthy MG, Nguyen TN. Graft selection in reconstruction of the anterior cruciate ligament. *J Bone Joint Surg Br*. 2001;83(5):625-634.

14. Tadokoro K, Matsui N, Yagi M, Kuroda R, Kurosaka M, Yoshiya S. Evaluation of hamstring strength and tendon regrowth after harvesting for anterior cruciate ligament reconstruction. *Am J Sports Med.* 2004;32(7):1644-1650.
15. Tashiro T, Kurosawa H, Kawakami A, Hikita A, Fukui N. Influence of medial hamstring tendon harvest on knee flexor strength after anterior cruciate ligament reconstruction. A detailed evaluation with comparison of single- and double-tendon harvest. *Am J Sports Med.* 2003;31(4):522-529.
16. Aglietti P, Buzzi R, Zaccherotti G, De Biase P. Patellar tendon versus doubled semitendinosus and gracilis tendons for anterior cruciate ligament reconstruction. *Am J Sports Med.* 1994;22(2):211-217; discussion 217-218.
17. Hiemstra LA, Webber S, MacDonald PB, Kriellaars DJ. Knee strength deficits after hamstring tendon and patellar tendon anterior cruciate ligament reconstruction. *Med Sci Sports Exerc.* 2000;32(8):1472-1479.
18. Friis EA, Cooke FW, McQueen DA, Henning CE. Effect of bone block removal and patellar prosthesis on stresses in the human patella. *Am J Sports Med.* 1994;22(5):696-701.

WHEN DO YOU USE ALLOGRAFT TISSUES FOR PRIMARY ACL SURGERY?

Warren R. Dunn, MD, MPH

Introduction

I use an allograft when, after a lengthy discussion about potential options, the patient requests it. In my opinion, one cannot begin to discuss the topic of graft choice for primary anterior cruciate ligament (ACL) reconstruction without first including a brief discussion on informed consent because the answer to the question of graft choice arises from a broader dialogue, including the different types of graft options and their potential complications, which is an integral part of the informed consent process for primary ACL reconstruction.

Informed Consent

The purpose of informed consent is to respect patient autonomy and to enable patients to make decisions that reflect their values.[1] The principle of informed consent started in the early 1900s and has evolved over the years[2] and today reflects a process, not merely a written document. The process starts with the discussion between the physician and the patient/legal guardian and ends with the signing of the surgical consent document. While this may seem rather simple and obvious, the content and nature of the discussion is oftentimes suboptimal. The discussion should include an unbiased summary of the available evidence for the different graft choices, which we will discuss in more detail later in the chapter and in the subsequent chapter. Regardless of the content and nature of the informed consent discussion, patients will often unintentionally subvert this process by asking the surgeon to tell them which is the best graft choice. When this occurs, it can be tempting for the surgeon to advise the patients based on his or her preference. Surgeon preference, however, is not always evidence based and can stem from many things, including training or clinical experience. In the end, the surgeon should clearly state which information is based on evidence and which information is based on his or her preference.

Allografts

Although numerous graft options have been described in the literature, an in-depth discussion of the more common choices would be sufficient for the informed consent discussion and should include allografts in addition to central third patellar tendon and hamstring tendon autografts. An exception to this would be if the patient inquires about or the surgeon has experience with an alternative graft, such as the quadriceps tendon. In such cases, alternative grafts should also be included in the informed consent discussion.

Allografts have gained wider acceptance for a variety of procedures over the past 2 decades. According to the Centers for Disease Control and Prevention (CDC), the American Association of Tissue Banks (AATB) distributes approximately 1.5 million bone and tissue allografts annually in the United States.[3] Despite their increasing use, there is a paucity of good quality studies looking at outcomes. Currently, there are no randomized trials comparing fresh frozen allograft to autograft, whereas there are several level 1 studies showing similar outcomes between 2 commonly used autograft options: central third patellar tendon and hamstring tendon.[4] What little evidence is published on allografts not only suffers from weak study design but also from variation in the types of allograft material studied, sterilization techniques, and processing/storage methods. These methodological flaws make it difficult to determine best practices when it comes to the use of allografts.

Two of the main concerns surrounding the use of allografts are disease transmission and graft failure and thus should be discussed during the process of informed consent. Patients are often worried that they may catch a disease. One possible explanation for this may be the widespread media coverage of the fatal *Clostridium* transmission case in 2001. It turns out that this allograft came from a nonaccredited tissue bank, and the local AATB-accredited tissue bank declined the donor because the body had not been refrigerated for 19 hours. According to the AATB, the last reported case of disease transmission was in 2002 and was the result of a classic "window period"—the period after an infection has occurred but before an immune response can be detected with a lab test. As a result of this and other previous cases, all AATB-accredited tissue banks are now required to perform more sensitive testing in order to reduce the window period for disease transmission. As a result of this and other measures aimed at reducing the risk of disease transmission, I would recommend using a nonprofit tissue bank that is accredited by the AATB when the patient requests the use of an allograft. The AATB has standards for tissue processing that are typically higher than those set forth by the Food and Drug Administration (FDA).

In addition to disease transmission, graft failure is a concern related to the use of allografts. In the absence of good evidence demonstrating that allografts are associated with significantly higher graft failure compared to autografts, it seems reasonable to consider the use of an allograft provided that it is fresh frozen from an accredited tissue bank and has not been processed in a fashion that weakens the graft, such as high levels of irradiation used for deep contamination of tissue. However, it is important to keep in mind the fallacy often associated with lack of proof of the negative.

Conclusion

Despite the lack of randomized controlled trials directly comparing autografts and allografts, there are theoretical advantages to allografts, such as avoiding graft site morbidity and pain and shortened operative times. These advantages, however, must be weighed carefully against the distinct possibility of a higher graft failure rate. During the informed consent process, I try to convey these concepts to the patient in the context of the current best evidence on allografts. Whenever possible, I strive to make graft choice a shared decision that not only preserves the patient's autonomy but also incorporates his or her preferences.

References

1. Dunn WR, George MS, Churchill L, Spindler KP. Ethics in sports medicine. *Am J Sports Med.* 2007;35(5):840-844.
2. Bhattacharyya T, Yeon H, Harris MB. The medical-legal aspects of informed consent in orthopaedic surgery. *J Bone Joint Surg Am.* 2005;87:2395-2400.
3. Centers for Disease Control and Prevention. Frequently asked questions about tissue transplants. Available at: http://www.cdc.gov/ncidod/dhqp/tissueTransplantsFAQ.html. Accessed April 18, 2007.
4. Poolman RW, Abouali JA, Conter HJ, Bhandari M. Overlapping systematic reviews of anterior cruciate ligament reconstruction comparing hamstring autograft with bone-patellar tendon-bone autograft: why are they different? *J Bone Joint Surg Am.* 2007;89:1542-1552.

After an Acute ACL Injury in a Competitive Athlete, How Do You Manage the Patient in Preparation for Surgery?

Anne E. Colton, MD, and Charles A. Bush-Joseph, MD

In a competitive athlete, an anterior cruciate ligament (ACL) rupture can be a devastating injury. The anterior cruciate ligament is essential for knee stability in most athletic endeavors, specifically those that require cutting, pivoting, and jumping. It is important to reconstruct the ligament as soon as possible in order to minimize the time to return to play and maximize results. However, reconstruction of the ACL immediately following rupture has been shown to be associated with an increase in postoperative arthrofibrosis, slower return of quadriceps function, and range of motion loss[1,2] (Figure 9-1). These problems can be detrimental to the competitive athlete. To prevent this loss, Shelbourne and Faulk,[2] as well as Harner et al,[1] recommended waiting 21 to 28 days before reconstruction of a ruptured ACL. This waiting period allows for the subsidence of the inflammation, swelling, and resultant loss of motion. Using these principles, reoperation for motion loss after ACL surgery has gone from 12% to 14% to now less than 1%.

Rather than specifically mandate a time period prior to surgery, I prefer to look at the following parameters. It is imperative that the athlete regains full symmetric extension and 120 degrees of flexion prior to reconstruction. The knee should have little to no effusion. The patient should have strong quadriceps activity with normal or near normal gait pattern. Most times, I will send the patient shortly after injury to physical therapy to help maximize this effort. The therapist will utilize modalities such as cryotherapy, compression, and anti-inflammatory medications to reduce pain and swelling. In addition, attention must be focused on relieving the quadriceps inhibition that is present following this injury. Techniques such as closed-chain quadriceps exercises, straight leg raises, and electrical muscle stimulation can aid to recondition the quadriceps musculature.

Figure 9-1. Sixteen-year-old female with 22-degree flexion contracture 6 months after early ACL reconstruction performed 7 days postinjury. Patient required extensive arthroscopic lysis of adhesion to regain full extension.

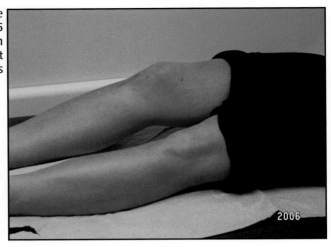

Restrictions must be reinforced and maintained during this preoperative period, such as avoiding cutting, pivoting, and jumping to prevent any instability events that could damage articular cartilage or menisci.

Once these parameters are achieved, I feel comfortable proceeding with ACL reconstruction. In some cases, this may occur rapidly within 1 to 2 weeks or it may take up to 6 to 8 weeks. However, I prefer to use this clinical criteria rather than a specific time frame when determining the timing of surgery.

In occasional rare instances in which patients are unable to regain full extension, the physician is responsible for ensuring that there is no mechanical cause such as a displaced meniscal tear or entrapped ligament stump. In those cases, the physician may proceed with arthroscopic debridement or meniscal repair and defer ACL reconstruction until motion improves.

References

1. Harner CD, Irrgang JJ, Paul J, Dearwater S, Fu FH. Loss of motion after anterior cruciate ligament reconstruction. *Am J Sports Med.* 1992;20:499-506.
2. Shelbourne KD, Foulk AD. Timing of surgery in anterior cruciate ligament tears on the return of quadriceps muscle strength after reconstruction using an autogenous patellar tendon graft. *Am J Sport Med.* 1995;23:686-689.

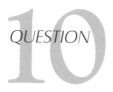
WHAT OPTIONS ARE AVAILABLE IN THE PATIENT WHO HAS A TIBIAL EMINENCE FRACTURE AVULSION (SKELETALLY MATURE, MIDDLE-AGED PATIENT)?

Anne E. Colton, MD, and Charles A. Bush-Joseph, MD

Tibial eminence fractures are more commonly seen in children and adolescents, as their ligaments are stronger and more durable than their bones, leading to failure. However, these fractures are sometimes seen in an adult population. In fact, Kendall et al[1] found that adult tibial spine fractures may be more common than previously thought. In their series, 60% of patients reviewed were adults.

Meyers and McKever[2] classified tibial spine fractures into 3 types based on their displacement. Zaricznyj[3] later added a fourth type:

I. Minimally displaced

II. Posterior hinge intact

III. Fragment completely separated

IV. Comminuted fragment ± rotation

Patients will present following an injury to their knee, much like the presentation of an ACL disruption: acutely swollen with a painful knee with limited range of motion. Aspiration of the knee will demonstrate hemarthrosis with marrow infiltration. X-rays obtained (Figure 10-1) will reveal the fracture, although displacement may not be easily discerned. It is important to acknowledge the presence of other injuries, including concomitant tibial plateau fractures, meniscal tears, and ligament disruptions, through physical examination, radiographs, and magnetic resonance imaging (MRI) evaluation.

Type I and II fractures are typically treated conservatively. Aspiration can help relieve the tense hemarthrosis that typically develops, allowing for reduction of the knee into extension. If reduction proves to be difficult, closed reduction under either general or intra-articular anesthesia is used. The patient is placed in a knee immobilizer for 4 to 6 weeks, allowing weight bearing as tolerated with crutches.

Figure 10-1. Anteroposterior (AP) and lateral x-rays of the knee reveal a tibial eminence fracture.

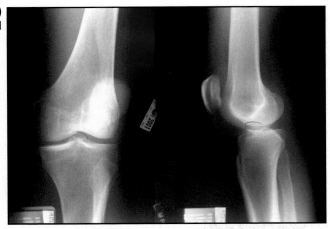

Figure 10-2. Arthroscopic photo of a tibial eminence fracture.

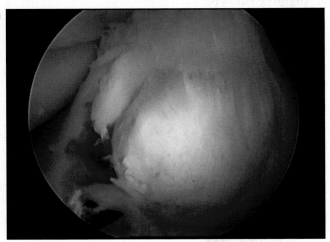

If the patient has a displaced tibial spine fracture, a type III or IV, or an irreducible type II, arthroscopic reduction and stabilization of the fracture is my preferred approach (Figure 10-2). For this procedure, the usual arthroscopic setup is utilized. A synovial resector is used to debride the fracture bed at the base of the tibial spine. Typically, a probe is used to reduce the fracture while another instrument, a probe or an anterior cruciate ligament (ACL) guide, maintains the reduction. A 0.062-inch K-wire is placed percutaneous through the midpatellar portal position to fix the reduced fragment. If the fragment is large enough, a 4.0-mm cannulated screw can be placed over this wire. However, if the fracture is comminuted, suture fixation is much more effective. This is accomplished by placing a Bunnell-type stitch through the ligament with heavy nonabsorbable suture (Figure 10-3). Again the K-wire is used, and an ACL guide is used to pass the suture from the anteromedial tibia, around the ligament, and back down through and out the anteromedial cortex of the tibia. The sutures are then tied over the bone bridge while the fracture is held reduced (Figure 10-4).

Postoperatively, the injury is treated much like an ACL reconstruction. The patient is weight bearing as tolerated in a knee brace, and rehabilitation is begun soon after the surgery, focusing on closed-chain quadriceps strengthening and range of motion exercises.

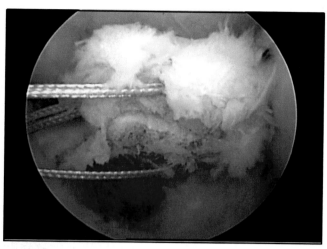

Figure 10-3. Tibial eminence with attached anterior cruciate ligament is shown with sutures placed before reduction.

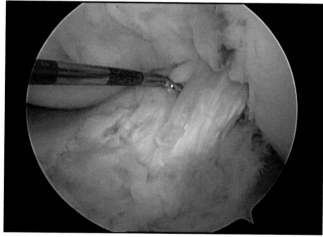

Figure 10-4. Reduced fracture is demonstrated.

In adult patients with comminuted fractures, the final option is delayed ACL reconstruction. A higher rate of stiffness has been reported in patients undergoing fixation of tibial eminence fractures. Secondly, some patients may have persistent laxity due to intrasubstance stretch injury within the ligament, which is not addressed by primary fixation. In older patients, delayed primary ACL reconstruction may provide a more reproducible result with lower complication rate compared to primary fixation.

References

1. Kendall NS, Hsu SYC, Chan K. Fracture of the tibial spine in adults and children. *J Bone Joint Surg Br.* 1992; 74:848-853.
2. Meyers MH, McKeever FM. Fracture of the intercondylar eminence of the tibia. *J Bone Joint Surg Am.* 1970; 52:1677-1684.
3. Zaricznyj B. Avulsion fracture of the tibial eminence: treatment by open reduction and pinning. *J Bone Joint Surg Am.* 1977;59:1111-1114.

Do You Prefer Endoscopic or 2-Incision Technique and Why?

James L. Carey, MD, and Kurt P. Spindler, MD

A systematic review of four prospective, randomized clinical trials (level I evidence) compared these 2 operative techniques.[1] Perioperative and outcome data were extracted from the original articles, including the following: operative time, length of hospital stay, activity level, instrumented laxity, range of motion, strength, pain, knee scores, and complications.[1] Two of the studies demonstrated that operative time and tourniquet time may be shorter using the endoscopic technique.[2,3] One study revealed a somewhat higher rate of return to activity and improved instrumented laxity in the rear-entry group as compared to the endoscopic group.[4] However, overall, these studies found no reproducible clinically relevant differences in subjective or objective data.[1] Therefore, a surgeon can choose either technique based on his or her preference.

We prefer the 2-incision technique for the following reasons. First, the rear-entry technique makes it difficult to place the graft too vertical or too anterior. This is due to the anatomy of the distal femur, the approach from the posterolateral aspect, and the curvature of the drill guide of the rear-entry system. Therefore, the 2 most common technical errors in anterior cruciate ligament (ACL) reconstruction (ie, the mistake in being too vertical or too anterior, Figures 11-1 and 11-2) are prevented.

Second, the harvested autograft bone-tendon-bone is appropriately length-matched to the tunnels. Thus, a bone block almost never fails to lie within a bony tunnel. This reproducibility in graft-tunnel matching yields reliable interference fixation.

Finally, and perhaps most importantly, the femoral tunnel is drilled independently of both the tibial tunnel and the anteromedial portal. This avoids the problem encountered when the angle of the tibial tunnel does not allow for proper placement of the graft, referenced to the over-the-top position and down the wall at 10 o'clock or 2 o'clock (Figures 11-3, 11-4, and 11-5). Likewise, an anteromedial portal can be problematic in an elongated notch (anterior to posterior) and/or narrow notch, preventing proper posterior placement of the femoral tunnel and risking damage to the medial femoral condyle.

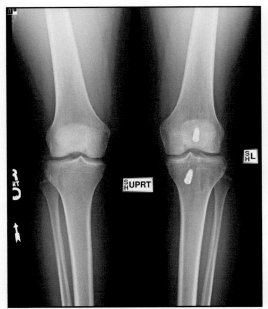

Figure 11-1. Bilateral standing knee x-rays reveal the common technical error of placing the graft too vertical and anterior—a "central cruciate reconstruction." This graft failed and the arthroscopy photos in the following figures were taken during the revision ACL reconstruction procedure.

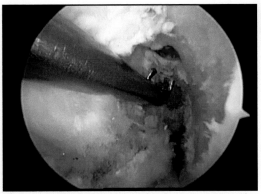

Figure 11-2. A 7-mm guide demonstrates the vertical and anterior placement of the prior femoral tunnel.

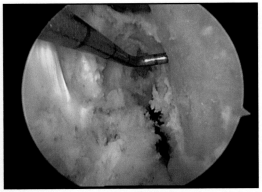

Figure 11-3. A probe illustrates the desired notch aperture of the new femoral tunnel, which is more posterior than the original tunnel and further down the wall, in the 2 o'clock position.

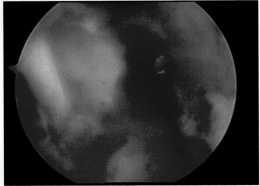

Figure 11-4. Using a rear-entry technique and a vector-orientating drill guide, the femoral tunnel is precisely drilled to the desired aperture point from outside to inside, independently of both the tibial tunnel and anteromedial portal.

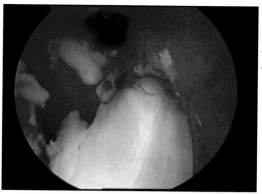

Figure 11-5. The final orientation of the graft more closely approximates the native ACL orientation and, consequently, provides more rotational stability than the previous vertically oriented graft.

References

1. George MS, Huston LJ, Spindler KP. Endoscopic versus rear-entry ACL reconstruction: A systematic review. *Clin Orthop Relat Res.* 2006;455:158-161.
2. Brandsson S, Faxen E, Eriksson BI, Sward L, Lundin O, Karlsson J. Reconstruction of the anterior cruciate ligament: comparison of outside-in and all-inside techniques. *Br J Sports Med.* 1999;33:42-45.
3. Gerich TG, Lattermann C, Fremerey RW, Zeichen J, Lobenhoffer HP. One- versus two-incision technique for anterior cruciate ligament reconstruction with patellar tendon graft: Results on early rehabilitation and stability. *Knee Surg Sports Traumatol Arthrosc.* 1997;5:213-216.
4. O'Neill DB. Arthroscopically assisted reconstruction of the anterior cruciate ligament. A prospective randomized analysis of three techniques. *J Bone Joint Surg.* 1996;78A:803-813.

How Do You Examine the Knee for Posterolateral Corner Injury Combined With ACL Injury?

Luke S. Oh, MD, and Thomas L. Wickiewicz, MD

Isolated posterolateral corner (PLC) injuries are rare (<2%), but there is a high incidence of PLC injuries in combination with anterior cruciate ligament (ACL) and/or posterior cruciate ligament (PCL) tears (43% to 80%). Therefore, patients with PLC injuries should be evaluated for concomitant injury to the cruciate ligaments. Conversely, for every patient who presents with what initially may appear to be just another routine ACL (or PCL) tear, a careful history and physical examination should be performed to evaluate for PLC injury in addition to cruciate injury. Beware that unrecognized PLC injury is a cause for failure in up to 50% of otherwise technically sound ACL reconstructions.

The first step in the evaluation of a possible PLC injury is to obtain a thorough history and to understand the mechanism of injury. The most common mechanisms for PLC injuries are (1) impact to the anteromedial aspect of the knee with the knee at or near full extension, (2) either contact or noncontact hyperextension injury, (3) varus load to a flexed knee, and (4) knee dislocation. When any of these injury mechanisms are reported, there should be a heightened clinical suspicion of PLC injury.[1] Patients will usually complain of pain in the posterolateral aspect of the knee, and some may also report paresthesias, numbness, or weakness from an associated common peroneal nerve injury. Patients frequently have functional instability when the knee is in extension. For example, the knee may give way into hyperextension during activities such as ascending and descending stairs or demonstrate instability with twisting, pivoting, or cutting maneuvers. Posterolateral rotatory instability (PLRI) is a term coined to describe posterior subluxation of the lateral tibial plateau that can occur with an external rotation torque in knees with pathologic laxity of the PLC. Symptoms of PLRI can occur acutely after severe injury, or they can develop insidiously after a relatively mild PLC injury.

During physical examination in the office, begin with an evaluation of the patient's standing alignment and gait. Important findings to note during the examination of the patient while standing include varus knee alignment, inability to stand with full knee extension, amount of discomfort while bearing weight, presence of quadriceps atrophy, and extent of swelling around the knee and of the extremity. Evaluation of gait may reveal the presence of an antalgic gait, hyperextension varus thrust, or footdrop. With a grade III LCL injury, the incidence of peroneal nerve injury is 12% to 29%.[2]

Next, with the patient sitting on the exam table, evaluate active knee range of motion (ROM), presence of a flexion contracture, and quad atrophy/weakness. Finally, with the patient supine, perform a careful neurovascular assessment before evaluating the knee with various stress examination maneuvers. Given that common peroneal nerve palsy and vascular injury are associated with PLC injuries sustained from higher energy mechanisms of injury, it is important to document the presence of any numbness/paresthesias on the dorsum of the foot, weakness with ankle dorsiflexion, and asymmetric distal pulses. If there is suspicion of a knee dislocation that had spontaneously reduced, an arteriogram may be appropriate.

Patients with significant effusion, flexion contracture, discomfort with terminal extension, and guarding secondary to pain or anxiety often find it more comfortable when their thigh is supported on a pillow while lying supine on an exam table. Placing a pillow under the thigh encourages the patient to relax, reduce guarding, and allows the surgeon to perform a meaningful examination of the knee. Moreover, a pillow under the thigh places the knee in approximately 30 degrees of flexion, which makes it ideal to perform a Lachman, varus/valgus stress, and tibial external rotation tests. While the patient is relaxed, the knee should be carefully examined for effusion, edema, ecchymosis, induration, and tenderness. Patients with acute PLC injury usually have tenderness over the posterolateral region of the knee, with tenderness localized over the fibular head or at the joint line in patients with arcuate or Segond fracture, respectively.[3] Positioning the knee in the FABER (flexed-abducted externally rotated) position is usually helpful in identifying an area of point tenderness in the posterolateral region of the knee.

According to Veltri and Warren,[4] the most useful tests for the diagnosis of posterolateral knee injury were the varus stress test at 0 and 30 degrees of flexion (Figure 12-1) and the prone external rotation test at 30 and 90 degrees of flexion (Figure 12-2). For the diagnosis of posterolateral instability, they utilized other tests such as the external-rotation recurvatum test (Figure 12-3) and the reverse pivot-shift test (Figure 12-4) in order to confirm their clinical impression. To increase accuracy, patients with a concomitant tear of the PCL should have any posterior subluxation reduced while the posterolateral aspect of the knee is evaluated. This can be achieved by having an assistant maintain the tibia in a reduced position while the patient is supine or by placing the patient in the prone position.

Tibial External Rotation Test

Also known as the "dial test," it can be performed with the patient either prone or supine. The prone position may be easier for documenting side-to-side differences in the thigh–foot angle. The test is performed at both 30 and 90 degrees of knee flexion, and

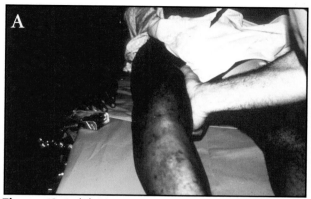

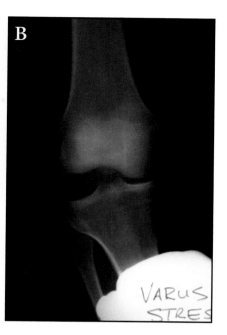

Figure 12-1. (A) Varus stress testing should be performed at 0 and 30 degrees of flexion. Varus instability at 30 degrees of flexion indicates injury to the lateral collateral ligament, whereas varus instability at both 0 and 30 degrees of flexion indicates injuries to the cruciate ligaments and the posterior capsule in addition to the lateral collateral ligament. (B) Varus stress radiograph demonstrating instability at full extension.

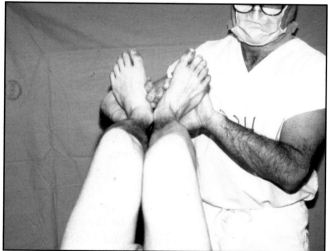

Figure 12-2. Tibial external rotation test, also known as the *dial test*, can be performed with the patient either prone or supine. The prone position may be easier for documenting side-to-side differences in the thigh–foot angle. The test is performed at both 30 and 90 degrees of knee flexion, and a positive test is noted when external rotation of the tibia exceeds that of the uninjured limb by 10 degrees or more. Increased external rotation at 30 degrees but not at 90 degrees indicates an isolated injury of the PLC, whereas increased external rotation at both angles suggests injury of both the PCL and PLC.

a positive test is noted when external rotation of the tibia exceeds that of the uninjured limb by 10 degrees or more. Increased external rotation at 30 degrees but not at 90 degrees indicates an isolated injury of the PLC, whereas increased external rotation at both angles suggests injury of both the PCL and PLC (see Figure 12-2). Testing is performed at both 30 and 90 degrees of flexion because the PCL is a secondary restraint against varus stress and external rotation.[5] At 90 degrees of flexion in a PCL-intact knee, all fibers of the PCL are taut and able to exert an effective secondary restraint against a varus moment or external rotation torque. At 30 degrees of knee flexion, only 10% to 15% of the PCL's fibers are taut and thus unable to effectively resist these motions.

Figure 12-3. External rotation recurvatum test is used to diagnose posterolateral rotatory instability with the knee in extension. It is performed by lifting the patient's legs by the great toes and noting any side-to-side differences in hyperextension, varus, and tibial external rotation.

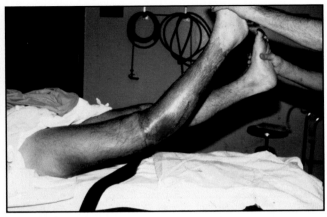

Figure 12-4. Reverse pivot-shift test is positive if there is a sensation of reduction when the flexed, externally rotated knee is extended with valgus stress.

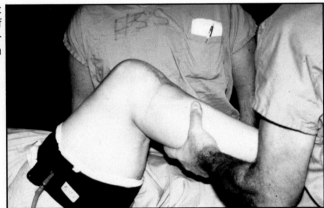

External Rotation Recurvatum Test

This test is used to diagnose PLRI with the knee in extension. It is performed by lifting the patient's legs by the great toes and noting any side-to-side differences in hyperextension, varus, and tibial external rotation (see Figure 12-3).

Reverse Pivot-Shift Test

This test is positive if there is a sensation of reduction when the flexed, externally rotated knee is extended with valgus stress (see Figure 12-4). The test may indicate injury of the PCL and the PLC, but it may be positive in up to 35% of normal knees examined under anesthesia.

References

1. Maynard MJ, Deng X, Wickiewicz TL, Warren RF. The popliteofibular ligament. Rediscovery of a key element in posterolateral stability. *Am J Sports Med.* 1996;24(3):311-316.
2. Covey DC. Injuries of the posterolateral corner of the knee. *J Bone Joint Surg Am.* 2001;83:106-118.
3. Seebacher JR, Inglis AE, Marshall JL, Warren RF. The structure of the posterolateral aspect of the knee. *J Bone Joint Surg Am.* 1982;64:536-541.
4. Veltri DM, Warren RF. Anatomy, biomechanics, and physical findings in posterolateral knee instability. *Clin Sports Med.* 1994;13:599-614.
5. Gollehon DL, Torzilli PA, Warren RF. The role of the posterolateral and cruciate ligaments in the stability of the human knee: a biomechanical study. *J Bone Joint Surg Am.* 1987;69:233-242.

SECTION II

INTRAOPERATIVE
QUESTIONS

WHAT DO YOU DO IF YOU DROP THE GRAFT ON THE FLOOR?

Mathew Busam, MD, and Bernard R. Bach, Jr., MD

Great care must be taken to avoid contamination during harvest and or preparation of the graft for anterior cruciate ligament (ACL) reconstruction. Our protocol emphasizes that the surgeon who harvests the graft personally walks the tissue to the back table to reduce the risk of dropping the graft. Handing off of a freshly harvested graft to other members of the surgical team for preparation simply increases the likelihood dropping the graft. With this protocol, the senior author has not dropped any grafts in over 20 years of practice, including more than 1700 knee ligament procedures. Careful attention must be paid during preparation on the back table as well. The fully prepared graft is placed in a marked kidney basin. All operative personnel are informed to prevent the graft from being inadvertently passed off the sterile field (Figure 13-1). When the graft is brought to the operative field for graft placement, if it is wrapped in a laparotomy sponge, theoretically the only contaminated portion would be the sutures extending beyond the sponge if the graft were dropped.

If the graft is dropped, the salvage falls into one of several possible categories, namely cleaning the graft, using an alternative graft (auto or allograft), or stopping the procedure and completing the surgery at another time with a different graft.

One study showed a 58% rate of positive culture when the graft was dropped and left on the operating room floor for 15 s. Molina et al have shown that a 90-s soak in chlorhexadine gluconate is the most effective method to resterilize the graft (Table 13-1).[1]

Another report found that a 30-min soak in 4% chlorhexadine followed by a 30-min soak in triple antibiotic solution (gentamicin, clindamycin, polymixin), followed by sterile saline wash was 100% effective in sterilizing contaminated rabbit patellar tendon grafts. In that same study, 10% povidone-iodine was 100% ineffective, as was triple antibiotic soak used in isolation.[2]

Figure 13-1. Clinical photo of graft conspicuously marked and placed safely on the back table.

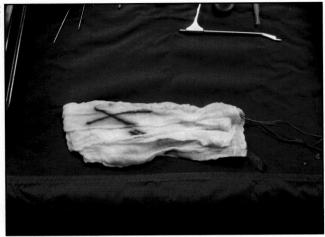

Table 13-1

Sterilizing Effectiveness on Bacterial Cultures

Sterilizing Agent	*Rate of Positive Culture (%)*
Chlorhexadine gluconate	2
Bacitracin and polymyxin	6
Povidone-iodine	24

A survey of sports medicine specialists found that most would choose cleansing the graft to manage the problem of a dropped graft. Forty-three surveyed surgeons reported having cleansed a contaminated graft and none reported postoperative infections.[3]

Another option is choosing an alternative graft. This requires preoperative consent from the patient or intraoperative consent from a family member and may be problematic for a patient who expects one graft type but ends up with another. Some surgeons routinely consent their patients for the use of an allograft should the autograph become contaminated or otherwise compromised. Again, if this option is selected, preoperative discussion with the patient is best because cultural or religious beliefs may preclude the use of cadaveric tissue.

Our preference would be cleansing the graft using a 30-min soak in 4% chlorhexadine gluconate followed by lavage with sterile saline, then another 30-min soak in triple antibiotic solution (0.1% gentamicin, 0.1% clindamicin, 0.05% polymyxin) and another sterile saline wash. Washing the chlorhexadine is crucial because chlorhexadine-induced chondrolysis has been reported.[4] While this protocol is time consuming, it has solid scientific backing and would allow one to proceed with the same graft as planned preoperatively. One could consider a course of postoperative antibiotics, although we would refrain from this as it would likely only mask an underlying infection, delaying its definitive treatment. In addition, we recommend full disclosure to the patient regarding the incident and the low likelihood of any residual difficulties.

References

1. Molina ME, Nonweiller DE, Evans JA, DeLee JC. Contaminated anterior cruciate ligament grafts: the efficacy of 3 sterilization agents. *Arthroscopy.* 2000;16:373-378.
2. Goebel ME, Drez D Jr, Heck SB, Stoma MK. Contaminated rabbit patellar tendon grafts: in vivo analysis of disinfecting methods. *Am J Sports Med.* 1994;22:387-391.
3. Izquierdo R Jr, Cadet ER, Bauer R, Stanwood W, Levine WN, Ahmad CS. A survey of sports medicine specialists investigating the preferred management of contaminated anterior cruciate ligament grafts. *Arthroscopy.* 2005;21:1348-1353.
4. Van Huyssteen AL, Bracey DJ. Chlorhexadine and chondrolysis in the knee. *J Bone Joint Surg Br.* 1999;81-B:995-996.

How Do You Manage a Posterior Wall Blowout Created Inadvertently at the Time of Surgery?

Matthew T. Provencher, MD, LCDR, MC, USN, and Nikhil N. Verma, MD

Optimal tunnel placement in anterior cruciate ligament (ACL) reconstruction remains critical for success. When investigating the causes of ACL reconstruction failure, although the overall causes are often multifactorial, graft malposition due to an incorrectly placed femoral tunnel is frequently described. In those cases where technical error in placement of the femoral tunnel has been demonstrated, the femoral tunnel is usually anterior and more vertical than the ACL femoral footprint.[1-4] Upon assessment of the best available literature, Beynnon et al[2] felt that the ideal placement of the femoral tunnel is along a line parallel to Blumensaat's line just posterior to the normal center of ACL attachment at the 10 o'clock position (left knee) or 2 o'clock position (right knee), without violating the posterior cortex. This is based on studies[5,6] that demonstrated increased clinical laxity[5] and graft impingement[6] with an anteriorly placed graft, even just 2 mm anterior to the normal center of ACL attachment.[4] However, when trying to achieve this construct, the posterior cortex of the femur may be violated by the drill, and the result is posterior wall blowout.

The best way to manage posterior wall blowout is prevention through careful intra-operative planning and calculation (Table 14-1). Several points should be kept in mind to avoid posterior wall blowout (Table 14-2):

* The minimum recommended distance of 1.5 to 2 mm of posterior back wall should be calculated into the femoral offset guide and added to the tunnel radius.

* Choose the correct femoral offset guide. For example, for an 8-mm graft, a 2-mm back wall will be obtained with a 6-mm offset guide, and for a 10-mm graft, a 1-mm back wall will result with a 6-mm over-the-top guide. These can be altered to obtain different back wall length if desired.

Table 14-1

Basic Bailout Strategies for Posterior Wall Blowout

Surgical Strategy to Manage Posterior Wall Blowout	*Special Equipment To Consider Having on Hand*
Extra-articular reconstruction (over-the-top fixation)[10]	Over-the-top guide system
Two-incision technique [1,2,5,6,12]	Rear-entry (or equivalent) femoral guide
Suspension fixation [4,11]	EndoButton system (4.5-mm drill and implants), strong suture (#5 Ethibond or equivalent)
Improve coronal trajectory if adequate bone remaining laterally down cortex to allow divergent tunnel; consider medial portal technique to redrill	Medial portal technique: separate medial femoral portal for drilling; knee flexion at 120 degrees, ensure divergent tunnel, watch femoral cartilage when passing femoral drill

Table 14-2

Pearls to Avoid Blowout

- We recommend that the femoral tunnel be drilled at 90 to 95 degrees of flexion.
- Appropriately sized over-the-top guide. Do the math for your over-the-top guide (OTG) at the conclusion of graft preparation.
- Coronal trajectory: vertical tunnel with less of a posterior wall centrally than laterally down the notch
- Test femoral drill pattern by "scoring" a footprint on the lateral femoral cortex, pulling the femoral drill back, and checking amount of posterior wall

∗ Knee flexion angle during femoral drilling. A femoral tunnel that is drilled at less than 80 degrees of knee flexion risks posterior wall blowout, especially of the most distal and posterior femoral cortex. The drill will penetrate the posterior cortex soon after entry into the femoral tunnel.[3,4]

∗ Once the guide pin is in place and the correct femoral drill is chosen, use the femoral drill to "score" a footprint on the inner aspect of the notch, back up the drill, and check to ensure that there is sufficient back wall (Figure 14-1).[3,7,8] Drilling can be resumed if there is sufficient back wall; otherwise, reposition the guide wire.

In either the primary or revision situation, if posterior wall blowout is encountered, one must have sufficiently rehearsed strategies to overcome this problem. If there is only a small amount of posterior wall involved (2 to 3 mm in depth), we recommend probing the tunnel to ensure integrity and proceeding with interference screw fixation as planned.[7] However, if there is more significant posterior wall blowout, interference screw fixation is not adequate. Thus, we recommend conversion to either a 2-incision technique[1,8-11] using a suitable rear-entry (or other type) femoral guide and drilling another tunnel, divergent

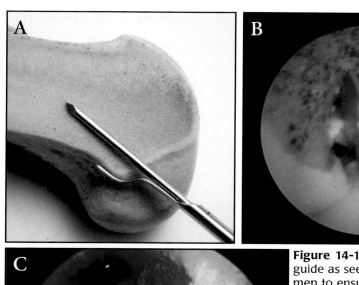

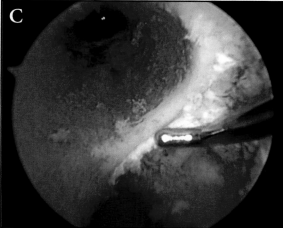

Figure 14-1. (A) The over the top guide as seen on a cadaveric specimen to ensure that there is no posterior wall blowout. (B) The acorn reamer is inserted only a few millimeters and then withdrawn to ensure that there is adequate back wall as shown in C.

from the first usually more lateral down the femoral notch, or conversion to suspension or cross-pin fixation with possible aperture fixation supplementation.[7,12] We recommend the suspension fixation because the cross-pin fixation systems require tunnel integrity for optimal performance. It is relatively easy to convert to a suspension fixation—the femoral tunnel is drilled sufficiently to accommodate the suspension device (EndoButton, Smith & Nephew, Andover, MA) and allow for the flipping of the button over the lateral femoral cortex. The original bone-tendon-bone (BTB) graft can be retained and large sutures secured to the bone plug, tendon (whipstitch), and EndoButton for a secure fixation. The suture length between the EndoButton and the bone plug has to accommodate the tunnel depth and flip required for setting the EndoButton against the lateral cortex.

In addition to suspension fixation, an over-the-top fixation has also been described[4] in cases of posterior blowout. A second incision is made on the lateral aspect of the femur, just proximal to the epicondyle and the iliotibial band is incised. The posterolateral aspect of the femur is exposed, and a window is created to the intercondylar notch by penetrating the intermuscular septum. The graft can then be secured to the femoral cortex via screw or staples.

One can avoid posterior wall blowout through sound operative principles such as notch preparation, correct tunnel placement, knee flexion at 90 degrees or greater when drilling the femoral tunnel, and use of a correct over the top guide. However, if posterior wall blowout is encountered, familiarization with these techniques, as well as having the equipment on hand to perform these bailout surgeries, is mandatory when one is performing ACL reconstructive surgery.

References

1. Azar FM, Arthur S. Complications of anterior cruciate ligament reconstruction. *Tech Knee Surg.* 2004;3(4):238-250.
2. Beynnon BD, Johnson RJ, Abate JA, Fleming BC, Nichols CE. Treatment of anterior cruciate ligament injuries, part 2. *Am J Sports Med.* 2005;33(11):1751-1767.
3. Johnson D. Techniques in knee surgery anterior cruciate ligament reconstruction. *Tech Knee Surg.* 2006; 5(2):107-120.
4. Lahav A, Burks R. Evaluation of the failed ACL reconstruction. *Sports Med Arthrosc Rev.* 2005;13(1):8-16.
5. Good L, Odensten M, Gillquist J. Sagittal knee stability after anterior cruciate ligament reconstruction with a patellar tendon strip. A two-year follow-up study. *Am J Sports Med.* 1994;22(4):518-523.
6. Khalfayan EE, Sharkey PF, Alexander AH, Bruckner JD, Bynum EB. The relationship between tunnel placement and clinical results after anterior cruciate ligament reconstruction. *Am J Sports Med.* 1996;24(3):335-341.
7. Creighton R, Bach B Jr. Revision anterior cruciate ligament reconstruction with patellar tendon allograft. *Sports Med Arthrosc Rev.* 2005;13(1):38-45.
8. Gomoll A, Bach B Jr. Managing tunnel malposition and widening in revision anterior cruciate ligament surgery. *Operat Tech Sports Med.* 2006;14:36-44.
9. Azar FM. Revision anterior cruciate ligament reconstruction. *Instr Course Lect.* 2002;51:335-342.10.
   Flik K, Bach B Jr. Anterior cruciate ligament reconstruction using a two-incision arthroscopy-assisted technique with patellar tendon autograft. *Tech Orthop.* 2005;20(4):372-376.
11. Wupperman P, Spindler K. Revision ACL surgery using a two-incision technique. *Sports Med Arthrosc Rev.* 2005;13(1):32-37.
12. Prodromos C, Joyce B. Endobutton fixation for hamstring anterior cruciate ligament reconstruction: surgical technique and results. *Tech Orthop.* 2005;20(3):233-237.

How Do You Manage the Hamstring Autograft That Is Prematurely Amputated During Graft Harvest?

Robert H. Brophy, MD, and Riley J. Williams, III, MD

When using a hamstring autograft for anterior cruciate ligament (ACL) reconstruction, the strongest construct is the quadrupled gracilis (GR)-semitendinosis (ST) graft.[1,2] This graft construct relies upon the doubling of each tendon limb, around a post, to create a four-stranded graft that passes through the articular space. Grafts are typically obtained by isolating these tendons at their tibial insertion at the pes anserinus expansion. During graft harvest, care must be taken to avoid premature amputation of each of these tendons. Such a complication may result in there being an inadequate amount of autograft tissue remaining for ACL reconstruction. As such, the harvesting portion of this case remains its most critical step. Unfortunately, the premature amputation of one or both of these tendons will occur with even the most skilled surgeons at the helm. The surgeon should take a three-tiered approach to this complication, starting with prevention, progressing to salvage, and finally substitution.

Obviously, prevention is the preferred approach for dealing with any complication. In the case of premature amputation of the hamstrings, understanding the anatomy is the key to avoiding this setback.[3] The most likely sources of difficulty when using the tendon stripper are the fascial bands and accessory insertions commonly found at the distal aspect of the ST and GR tendons proximal to the pes; these bands typically diverge and insert on the fascia of the medial gastrocnemius muscle. Failure to release these bands may cause the tendon stripper to transect the primary tendon as the device is advanced into the distal thigh. These fascial bands are usually located 8 to 10 cm proximal to the pes insertion. The major accessory insertion (associated with the ST tendon) usually diverges from the tendon 5.5 cm (range 4.5 to 8 cm) proximal to the pes and typically inserts 3 cm distal to the inferior border of the conjoined tendon insertion site.[4] Up to 5 accessory insertions may be encountered.[3] The surgeon must be aware of these fascial bands and take great care to identify them by inspection and palpation. Band release should be done

Figure 15-1. Salvage technique when gracilis is prematurely amputated.

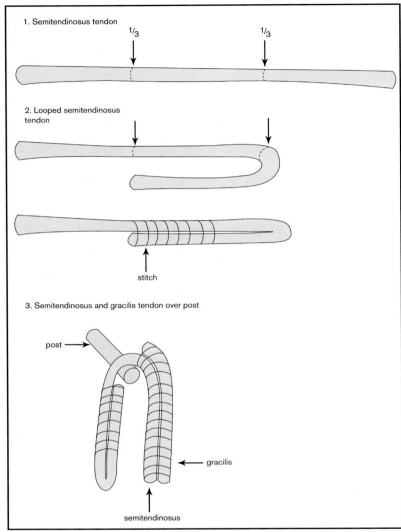

1. Semitendinosus tendon

¹/₃   ¹/₃

2. Looped semitendinosus tendon

stitch

3. Semitendinosus and gracilis tendon over post

post

gracilis

semitendinosus

under direct vision using surgical scissors prior to passing the tendon stripper. During the harvesting maneuver, if advancement of the stripper requires great effort or force during the first 5 to 20 cm, the surgeon should remove the device and inspect the tendon thoroughly for the described fascial bands.

Once amputation of the hamstrings has occurred, the option for salvage depends on which tendon is amputated. If the gracilis is cut, the semitendinosis can be divided into thirds and looped back upon itself such that a triple-limbed tendon graft is created. The remaining gracilis tendon, if salvageable, can be combined with this tripled semitendinosis graft to construct a quadrupled graft with three limbs from the semitendinosus and one limb from the gracilis (Figure 15-1). Such a graft construct can easily reach 8 to 9 mm of diameter due to the inherent bulk of the ST. The options are more limited if the ST tendon is amputated. In this case, one can attempt to triple-loop the gracilis as described for the semitendinosis, but the GR tendon tends to be small and may not provide the surgeon with adequate tissue for a suitable ACL graft. At best this construct is usually very small (around 6 mm diameter or less), which may not be sufficient to warrant its use in reconstruction.

In cases where the salvaged GR-ST tendon graft is inadequate due to its small size, the surgeon should move to substitution. The authors recommend that the surgeon move to a soft-tissue allograft construct in these cases. A tibialis anterior allograft is a strong, bulky graft that is easily substituted for the hamstring construct. However, the surgeon may opt to use the ipsilateral patellar tendon, contralateral hamstring tendons, or other allograft tissue sources, including Achilles tendon allograft or patellar tendon allograft. This choice is left to the experience and preference of the operating surgeon. The authors strongly recommend that alternative graft options should be discussed with the patient prior to surgery, since an alternative graft may be necessary for a number of reasons, including insufficient hamstring tendon size, graft contamination, or graft amputation. From the surgeon's perspective, use of the tibialis anterior allograft is advantageous because the tibial and femoral fixation that had been planned for the quadrupled hamstring can also be used with the tibialis anterior graft. In addition, use of the tibialis anterior graft avoids the potential donor site morbidity associated with violation of the knee extensor mechanism (patellar tendon autograft), which presumably contributed to the choice of a hamstring ACL graft in the first place. Patient preference, however, may preclude the use of allograft. In these cases, autograft patellar tendon graft or contralateral hamstring autograft would be preferable. The take-home message here is that for most hamstring autograft ACL procedures, the surgeon should always discuss alternative graft options to facilitate seamless intraoperative decision making.

References

1. Hamner DL, Brown CH Jr, Steiner ME, Hecker AT, Hayes WC. Hamstring tendon grafts for reconstruction of the anterior cruciate ligament: biomechanical evaluation of the use of multiple strands and tensioning techniques. *J Bone Joint Surg Am*. 1999;81:549-557.
2. Simonian PT, Williams RJ, Deng XH, Wickiewicz TL, Warren RF. Hamstring and patellar tendon graft response to cyclical loading. *Am J Knee Surg*. 1998;11:101-105.
3. Solman CG Jr, Pagnani MJ. Hamstring tendon harvesting. Reviewing anatomic relationships and avoiding pitfalls. *Orthop Clin North Am*. 2003;34:1-8.
4. Pagnani MJ, Warner JJ, O'Brien SJ, Warren RF. Anatomic considerations in harvesting the semitendinosus and gracilis tendons and a technique of harvest. *Am J Sports Med*. 1993;21:565-571.

16

How Would You Manage the Situation of Graft Amputation During Interference Screw Placement With a Patellar Tendon Graft?

Brian Kerr, MD, and Eric C. McCarty, MD

Careful attention to detail when placing interference screws helps to avoid potential complications, specifically graft amputation. During femoral interference screw placement, we carefully observe the tendinous portion of the graft just inferior to the bone plug. If this area begins to rotate, we are in danger of lacerating the graft and make adjustments accordingly.[1]

If graft laceration does occur, whether through bone, at the tendon-bone junction, or through soft-tissue planes, one's options are limited. The amount of remaining graft must be carefully examined to determine whether the graft itself is salvageable. If not, the operative plan can shift to an alternate graft source, with allograft replacement the most obvious and least invasive option—albeit expensive. Consideration can be given to using the contralateral graft choice, either patellar tendon or hamstring from the opposite knee. If a second graft is utilized, we recommend temporarily scrubbing out of surgery to disclose the complication and discuss this new plan with the patient's family members. This is especially recommended if the decision is made to switch to an allograft source.

A thorough evaluation of the amputated segment can guide decision making if the graft is still viable. This should note how the bone plug is damaged or whether the graft is amputated at the tendon-bone interface. A plug broken in the longitudinal plane—rendering its diameter too small for adequate interference screw fixation—can be "piggybacked" to an additional bone plug.[2] This is accomplished by attaching the additional bone plug with suture through drill holes and allows for restoration of an adequately sized bone plug to be used with an interference screw (Figure 16-1). Alternatively, a whipstitch-type securing suture (Krackow, etc) can be placed through the soft tissue and

Figure 16-1. Attachment of additional bone to fractured bone plug for additional bone interference fixation.

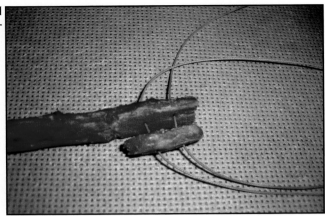

Figure 16-2. Short bone plug with Krackow stitches through tendon and bone plug.

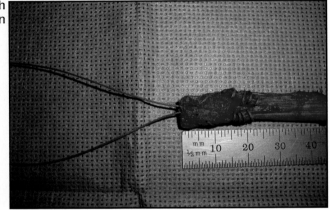

bony parts of the graft. This can be secured via suspension-type fixation, such as with an EndoButton (Smith & Nephew, Andover, MA). A bone-plug fractured transversely, that is, shortening of the bone plug, may not allow enough bone-screw contact length for adequate interference fixation, particularly if the remaining bone is shorter than 15 mm.[3] If this occurs, a Krackow stitch through tendon and bone with EndoButton fixation is our recommendation (Figure 16-2). For those surgeons familiar with 2-incision techniques and open lateral distal femoral fixation, these sutures can also be tied over a screw-and-washer post.[4]

If the amputation occurred at either the tendon-bone junction or in the tendon, we recommend removing the graft from the knee for thorough evaluation and removal of the amputated bone plug from the femoral tunnel. If adequate length remains, the graft may still be salvageable. If not, consideration again needs to be given to alternative graft choices. For grafts with adequate remaining length, a whipstitch-type suture should be used to secure the soft-tissue end. The graft should then be flipped, and the end with the remaining bone plug is placed into the femoral tunnel. The sutured end of the graft can then be secured to the tibia using preferred soft-tissue fixation, such as posts or screw and spiked washers.[2] With this method, the amputated bone plug can then be placed into the tibial tunnel over the secured graft, acting as bone graft for additional fixation. Alternatively, secondary fixation with a bioabsorbable screw in the tibial tunnel can be used.

We have found that certain techniques help us to prevent this very serious problem from occurring. Prior to passing the graft, we prefer to place a notch in the anterior portion of the femoral tunnel where we expect to place the interference screw. This can be done with commercially available notching instruments, but we use the interference screwdriver for this purpose, usually to a depth of 10 mm. By doing this, we facilitate guide wire and screw placement. Prior to screw placement, we place the knee in maximum flexion to minimize the chance for screw divergence. During placement of the screw, we pull continuous tension on the tibial-side graft sutures to prevent femoral plug advancement and rotation. If undue resistance to screw advancement is noted, we stop to reevaluate our technique and the direction of the screw relative to the bone block and femoral tunnel. Commercially available graft protectors may also be utilized to decrease the chance for injury.

References

1. D'Amato MJ, Bach BR. Anterior cruciate ligament injuries in the adult. In: DeLee JC, Drez D, Miller MD, eds. *Orthopaedic Sports Medicine*. Philadelphia, PA: Saunders; 2003:2012-2067.
2. Cain LE, Gillogly SD, Andrews JR. Management of intraoperative complications associated with autogenous patellar tendon graft anterior cruciate ligament reconstruction. *Instr Course Lect*. 2003;52:359-367.
3. Schock H, Freedman KB. Intraoperative complications: graft fixation problems. In Freedman KB, ed. *AAOS Monograph Complications in Orthopaedics: Anterior Cruciate Ligament Surgery*. Rosemont, IL: AAOS; 2005:9-19.
4. Dalton J, Harner C. Surgical techniques to correct nonanatomic femoral tunnels. *Oper Tech Sports Med*. 1998;6:83-90.

WHAT TRICKS DO YOU HAVE TO AVOID CREATION OF A "VERTICAL" TUNNEL WHEN DRILLING A TRANSTIBIAL TUNNEL?

Luke S. Oh, MD, and Thomas L. Wickiewicz, MD

A vertical graft may provide stability to anterior tibial translation but provides little rotational stability. Patients with a vertical graft will demonstrate a persistent pivot shift and remain functionally unstable. Therefore, the current recommendation is to place the femoral tunnel further down the lateral wall from the traditional 11 o'clock and 1 o'clock positions to the 10 o'clock and 2 o'clock positions.[1] When using the transtibial tunnel technique, a vertical femoral tunnel is a result of a vertical tibial tunnel because reaming the femoral tunnel is constrained by the tibial tunnel. Therefore, the trick to avoiding a vertical femoral tunnel is to create an appropriately placed tibial tunnel. A vertical graft may result if the tibial tunnel is placed too posterior or if the starting hole for the tibial tunnel is too lateral (closer to midline).

A tibial tunnel may end up too posterior in cases where the surgeon "cheats" the reamer to exit a bit more posteriorly inside the knee in order to ensure avoidance of anterior graft impingement and loss of extension. A posterior tibial tunnel makes it difficult to create a starting point for the femoral tunnel in the desired orientation and position on the clock-face. This usually results in a more centrally placed and vertically oriented femoral tunnel (Figure 17-1). In order to avoid a posterior tibial tunnel, the intra-articular positioning of the anterior cruciate ligament (ACL) tibial tunnel guide should be carefully scrutinized under arthroscopic visualization. In the coronal plane, place the knee in 90 degrees of flexion and assess the relationship of the tip of the tibial guide to the tibial spines, posterior cruciate ligament (PCL), and side wall of the intercondylar notch. The tip of the tibial guide should be placed between the tibial spines and lateral to the PCL. In the sagittal plane, the tip of the tibial guide should be placed at the junction of the anterior one-third and middle one-third of the ACL footprint. We prefer this method compared to placing the tibial guide 7 mm anterior to the PCL as recommended by Morgan et al because the number of millimeters may vary slightly depending on the size of the footprint.[2]

Figure 17-1. Plain radiographs of a knee with persistent pivot shift and rotational instability after ACL reconstruction. On the anteroposterior (AP) x-ray, the position of the graft is vertical. On the lateral x-ray, note that the tibial tunnel is posterior. When using the transtibial technique, a posterior tibial tunnel makes it difficult to create a starting point for the femoral tunnel in the desired orientation and position on the clockface. This usually results in a more centrally placed and vertically oriented femoral tunnel. (Radiographs courtesy of Bernard R. Bach, Jr., MD.)

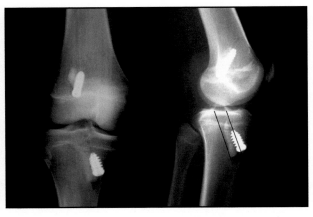

Figure 17-2. Arthroscopy confirmed that the tibial tunnel was misplaced too posteriorly. The intra-articular position of the tibial tunnel should be at the junction of the anterior one-third and middle one-third of the ACL footprint. The posterior edge of the anterior horn of the lateral meniscus (probe) can be used as a reference point for the position of the tibial tunnel in the sagittal plane. (Photograph courtesy of Bernard R. Bach, Jr., MD.)

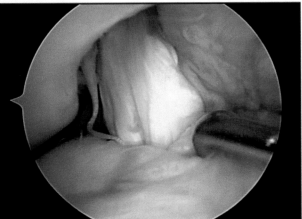

Remember that the native ACL has a broad insertion (19 to 23 mm) that flares anteromedially on the tibia. If the tibial tunnel is placed too anteriorly in the remnant of the broad insertion of the native ACL, the graft will likely cause roof impingement. As an additional intra-articular anatomic reference for accurate placement of the tibial guide in the sagittal plane, the tip of the tibial guide should be at the level of the posterior edge of the anterior horn of the lateral meniscus[3] (Figure 17-2).

Once the desired intra-articular position of the tibial guide has been identified, then the appropriate position of the alignment rod in the handle of the tibial guide needs to be determined. Since the native ACL has an oblique orientation as it traverses across the knee, the handle of the tibial guide should be appropriately supinated or pronated in order to mimic the anatomic obliquity of the ACL. In order to replicate the anatomic obliquity, the position of the tibial guide should be critically evaluated by arthroscopic and direct visualization. It should be noted that using the "N + 7" rule to determine the angle for the ACL tibial guide results in a tendency to rest the handle of the guide on the bone too anteriorly (closer to midline). Let the guide fit to the knee, not the knee to the guide. The position of the alignment rod on the tibia should be at the lateral-most edge of the medial collateral ligament (MCL) insertion. If you drop an imaginary plumb line from the anteromedial arthroscopic portal, the alignment rod should either be directly inferior or slightly medial. As a general rule, if the alignment rod on the proximal metaphysis is lateral (closer to midline) to the anteromedial portal, there is a risk of drilling a vertical tibial tunnel.[3]

After a guide wire has been placed through the appropriately positioned alignment rod, this allows for another opportunity to critically scrutinize the obliquity prior to reaming the tibial tunnel. Magnetic resonance imaging (MRI) studies have demonstrated that the coronal angle of the native ACL is between 63 and 71 degrees and that the normal sagittal angle is between 45 and 55 degrees.[4,5] Ideally, the guide pin should exit the tibia in between the tibial spines approximately 7 mm anterior to the PCL and at the level of the posterior margin of the anterior horn of the lateral meniscus. The tip of the guide wire should then be able to reach the 10 o'clock position on the femur for a right knee (2 o'clock position for a left knee) and 6 mm anterior to the back wall of the femur for a 10-mm graft. If this is not achievable, then the trajectory of the tibial tunnel should be changed. In certain cases, changing the trajectory of the tibial tunnel is not desirable; for example, during a revision ACL reconstruction with a preexisting enlarged tibial tunnel. In these situations, the surgeon should be prepared to abandon the transtibial technique and consider other methods to create a desirable femoral tunnel. Options include using an accessory anteromedial portal that allows drilling of a femoral tunnel in the desired position or using a 2-incision technique that employs either a Hewson guide or an Arthrex Retrodrill.

After the tibial tunnel is drilled in the desired orientation, insert the size-specific femoral aimer that corresponds to the size of the graft. Adjust knee flexion until the tip of the aimer is placed in the over-the-top position at 10 o'clock for a right knee or 2 o'clock for a left knee. Rotate the aimer away from the PCL approximately 30 degrees in order to prevent the femoral guide pin from skidding up the lateral wall during insertion. The femoral guide pin should form an inverted triangle with the PCL and roof. The cannulated acorn reamer should easily pass the PCL without touching it, and the posterior wall of the femoral tunnel should be 1 mm thick.

In summary, there are no real tricks to avoiding a vertical tunnel. Rather, meticulous technique is the key to avoiding misplaced tunnels.

References

1. Loh JC, Fukuda Y, Tsuda E, Steadman RJ, Fu FH, Woo SL. Knee stability and graft function following anterior cruciate ligament reconstruction: comparison between 11 o'clock and 10 o'clock femoral tunnel placement. 2002 Richard O'Connor Award Paper. *Arthroscopy.* 2003;19:297-304.
2. Morgan CD, Kalman VR, Grawl DM. Definitive landmarks for reproducible tibial tunnel placement in anterior cruciate ligament reconstruction. *Arthroscopy.* 1995:11(3):275-288.
3. Carson EW, Simonian PT, Wickiewicz TL, Warren RF. Revision anterior cruciate ligament reconstruction. *Instr Course Lect.* 1998;47:361-368.
4. Ayerza MA, Muscolo L, Costa-Paz M, Makino A, Rondon L. Comparison of sagittal obliquity of the reconstructed anterior cruciate ligament with native anterior cruciate ligament using magnetic resonance imaging. *Arthroscopy.* 2003;19(3):257-261.
5. Fujimoto E, Suman Y, Deie M, Yasumoto M, Kobayashi K, Ochi M. Anterior cruciate ligament impingement against the posterior cruciate ligament: diagnosis using MRI plus three-dimensional software. *Magn Reson Imaging.* 2004;22:1125-1129.

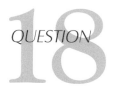

WHAT OPTIONS DO YOU HAVE AND HOW DO YOU MANAGE A CONSTRUCT MISMATCH WITH THE ENDOSCOPIC TECHNIQUE?

Matthew T. Provencher, MD, LCDR, MC, USN, and Nikhil N. Verma, MD

A construct mismatch is defined as a graft construct that is too long for the drilled tunnels and the graft protrudes from the tibial tunnel after femoral tunnel fixation. This problem is usually confined to autograft bone-patellar-bone (BTB) and allograft BTB reconstructions where optimal fixation of the bone block to both the femoral and tibial tunnels is desirable.[1-3] In the single-incision BTB anterior cruciate ligament (ACL) reconstruction, a graft-tunnel mismatch occurs if the tibial bone plug protrudes distally out of the tibial tunnel, making interference screw fixation difficult, and a tunnel that is too long makes distal fixation and femoral tunnel placement difficult.[3,4] Even with adequate preoperative planning and accurate intraoperative graft and tunnel measurements,[2,5,6] mismatch may still occur in a number of cases.[7]

Thus, the surgeon has to be adept at dealing with graft-tunnel mismatch in order to achieve optimal tibial fixation. Fortunately, there are a number of options to address graft-tunnel mismatch without compromising the biomechanical capabilities of the ACL graft. However, the best method to avoid mismatch is to employ operative planning techniques that will lead to accurate measurement of the graft and tunnel construct. Several principles have to be kept in mind when performing BTB ACL autograft reconstruction to minimize the chance of mismatch:

* Intra-articular ACL graft is approximately 19 to 22 mm.[2,6]

* Mean tibial bone tunnel length is approximately 48 to 53 mm when drilled with the guide at 55 degrees.[2]

* Mean tendon length is 41 to 49 mm;[2] this number is called "L."[6]

*   Sum of tibial tunnel and intra-articular ACL graft is approximately 68 to 74 mm.

*   The mean tibial tunnel length also increases with increasing tibial tunnel guide angle. Tunnels drilled at less than 45 degrees have a high risk on construct mismatch[2,3] (40 degrees guide yields approximately a 45-mm tunnel length).

*   Thus, the mean sum of the length of the ACL graft and tibial tunnel is approximately 68 to 75 mm.[2]

*   Due to the obliquity of the tunnel,[8] the measurements utilized to calculate length may be flawed when a bone plug protrudes that is not flush with the tibial surface but protrudes proximally and not distally at the tunnel orifice.

An "L + 7" rule has been suggested[6] to measure the tendon length (L) and add 7 mm, which will then be used to set the ACL drill guide (for example, a 45-mm graft would be a 52 degrees tunnel). However, this has been challenged due to potential mismatch with this rule,[7,8] and an "L + 10" rule has been suggested.[3] It has also been suggested that tunnels drilled at greater than 60 degrees may result in vertically oriented tunnels and are generally avoided.[3] Thus, if the intratendinous portion is greater than 50 mm, other methods to avoid mismatch must be employed. Thus, the risk of a mismatch is increased in intratendinous grafts greater than 50 mm and also with the use of allografts, which may be as high as 20%.[3]

Several methods are available to address graft-tunnel mismatch (Table 18-1). These can basically be divided into surgical management of the graft construct, the femoral tunnel, the tibial tunnel, or both tunnels.

On the tibial tunnel side, it has been shown that screw fixation in a porcine model could be reduced to 12.5-mm screw fixation with no biomechanical differences versus longer screws.[5] It would be prudent to have shorter interference screws available in a variety of diameters. Free bone plugs may also be press-fit into the tibial tunnel over the tendinous portion of the graft (remove the attached BTB plug). Even though the tibial bone block is removed, it has been shown in a bovine model that graft stiffness and ultimate load to failure are increased with a free bone block technique (90 N [Newtons]/mm; 669 N) versus screw-and-post fixation techniques (24 N/mm; 374 N).[3,9] Use of distal cortical tibial fixation devices, such as screw-post fixation and staples, has also been described;[3] however, graft tension and ability to maintain isometry are concerns. A variety of other bone grafting procedures have been described.[10,14]

On the femoral side, the most common mode of correction is to further recess the femoral bone plug. However, this technique is not without significant risk to graft integrity as laceration, premature amputation, posterior wall blowout, and graft abrasion at the tunnel edge are legitimate concerns.[3,4] Clinical results of this technique have been reported with no difference in KT-1000 arthrometry.[11] Also on the femoral side, the construct may be converted to a 2-incision technique. The graft is removed and an outside-in technique is utilized to drill the femoral tunnel, with the potential benefits of helping eliminate posterior wall blowout and tunnel mismatch.[3]

Our preferred methods for addressing mismatch deal with altering the ACL graft itself. In the setting of graft-tunnel mismatch, the graft is first externally rotated 180 degrees prior to tibial fixation.[3,13] Therefore, (1) this allows for the tibial screw to be placed against the cortical surface of the graft, (2) the graft is pushed more posterior to a more anatomic position, (3) cancellous-to-cancellous apposition of the bone plug is achieved, and (4) graft

Table 18-1

Methods of Intraoperative Correction of Graft-Tunnel Mismatch

Technique	Advantages	Disadvantages
Tibial Tunnel Correction		
Shorten tibial bone plug	Simple, need 12.5 mm of bone for adequate fixation[5]	Insufficient bone plug after resection
Free bone plug to the distal edge of graft after removing distal autograft plug completely and replacing, fix with interference screw[9]	Simple, need to be able to suture distal graft, may be used for graft or bone plug delamination	Healing and cyclic loading have not been studied
Autograft cancellous core of bone placed in tibial tunnel with interference screw[10]	Need to use coring reamer	Need harvest of cancellous core bone plug, might not be able to graft patella
Distal tibial cortical fixation	Staples, screw-post suspension fixation	Potential loss of graft isometry and graft tension problems[3]
Femoral Side Correction		
Femoral plug recession[11]	Need to identify screw and remove without transecting or lacerating graft	Graft laceration, isometry changes, posterior wall blow-out, inadequate fixation
Convert to 2-incision technique, remove graft, and utilize accessory lateral incision[3]	Avoids endoscopic complications (posterior wall blowout, mismatch)	Second incision necessary, vastus lateralis violation
ACL BTB Graft Correction		
Flip bone plug 180 degrees over itself, standard interference fixation[12]	Simple, graft has to be removed	Tunnel may not be able to accommodate increased girth of construct, bone may protrude intra-articularly
Rotate graft 540 degrees externally[13]	Mean shortening of 5.4 mm (11% of initial tendon length), increased ultimate failure strain, modulus decreased vs 180 degrees rotation construct	Difficulty to maintain graft tension on rotated graft, no evidence regarding cyclic loading of femoral-tibial construct
Rotation up to 630 degrees[1]	25% Shortening of graft, clinical stability retained at 1-year follow-up	Similar to previous

laceration is minimized. However, the graft is shortened by only 1 to 2 mm.[15] Thus, if mismatch occurs, the graft is rotated an additional 360 degrees for a total rotation of 540 degrees. This has been shown to shorten the graft 4 to 9 mm (or, about 10% of graft length)[13,15] while preserving modulus, yield stress, strain, and elasticity versus unrotated grafts. External rotation of the graft up to 630 degrees has also been described (shortens graft by about 25%).[1] The bone plug may also be flipped over itself[12] and subsequently fixed with an interference screw.

Preoperative planning and intraoperative calculation remain the best methods to avoid a graft-construct mismatch in ACL BTB autograft reconstruction. However, one should be ready to manage this graft-construct mismatch intraoperatively as it is not uncommon to encounter this problem.

References

1. Auge WK II, Yifan K. A technique for resolution of graft-tunnel length mismatch in central third bone-patellar tendon-bone anterior cruciate ligament reconstruction. *Arthroscopy.* 1999;15(8):877-881.
2. Denti M, Bigoni M, Randelli P, et al. Graft-tunnel mismatch in endoscopic anterior cruciate ligament reconstruction. Intraoperative and cadaver measurement of the intra-articular graft length and the length of the patellar tendon. *Knee Surg Sports Traumatol Arthrosc.* 1998;6(3):165-168.
3. Verma NN, Dennis MG, Carreira DS, Bojchuk J, Hayden JK, Bach BR Jr. Preliminary clinical results of two techniques for addressing graft tunnel mismatch in endoscopic anterior cruciate ligament reconstruction. *J Knee Surg.* 2005;18(3):183-191.
4. Hartman GP, Sisto DJ. Avoiding graft-tunnel mismatch in endoscopic anterior cruciate ligament reconstruction: a new technique. *Arthroscopy.* 1999;15(3):338-340.
5. Black KP, Saunders MM, Stube KC, Moulton MJ, Jacobs CR. Effects of interference fit screw length on tibial tunnel fixation for anterior cruciate ligament reconstruction. *Am J Sports Med.* 2000;28(6):846-849.
6. Olszewski AD, Miller MD, Ritchie JR. Ideal tibial tunnel length for endoscopic anterior cruciate ligament reconstruction. *Arthroscopy.* 1998;14(1):9-14.
7. Shaffer B, Gow W, Tibone JE. Graft-tunnel mismatch in endoscopic anterior cruciate ligament reconstruction: a new technique of intraarticular measurement and modified graft harvesting. *Arthroscopy.* 1993;9(6):633-646.
8. Kurzweil PR. Formula to calculate the length of the tibial tunnel with endoscopic ACL reconstruction to avoid graft-tunnel mismatch. *Arthroscopy.* 1999;15(1):115-117.
9. Novak PJ, Wexler GM, Williams JS Jr, Bach BR Jr, Bush-Joseph CA. Comparison of screw post fixation and free bone block interference fixation for anterior cruciate ligament soft tissue grafts: biomechanical considerations. *Arthroscopy.* 1996;12(4):470-473.
10. Fowler BL, DiStefano VJ. Tibial tunnel bone grafting: a new technique for dealing with graft-tunnel mismatch in endoscopic anterior cruciate ligament reconstruction. *Arthroscopy.* 1998;14(2):224-228.
11. Taylor DE, Dervin GF, Keene GC. Femoral bone plug recession in endoscopic anterior cruciate ligament reconstruction. *Arthroscopy.* 1996;12(4):513-515.
12. Barber FA. Flipped patellar tendon autograft anterior cruciate ligament reconstruction. *Arthroscopy.* 2000; 16(5):483-490.
13. Verma N, Noerdlinger MA, Hallab N, Bush-Joseph CA, Bach BR Jr. Effects of graft rotation on initial biomechanical failure characteristics of bone-patellar tendon-bone constructs. *Am J Sports Med.* 2003;31(5):708-713.
14. Mariani PP, Calvisi V, Margheritini F. A modified bone-tendon-bone harvesting technique for avoiding tibial tunnel-graft mismatch in anterior cruciate ligament reconstruction. *Arthroscopy.* 2003;19(1):E3.
15. Berkson E, Lee GH, Kumar A, Verma N, Bach BR Jr, Hallab N. The effect of cyclic loading on rotated bone-tendon-bone anterior cruciate ligament graft constructs. *Am J Sports Med.* 2006;34(9):1442-1449.

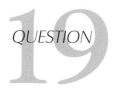

WHAT IS YOUR PREFERRED FIXATION METHOD FOR SOFT-TISSUE GRAFTS ON BOTH TIBIAL AND FEMORAL SIDES?

Seth C. Gamradt, MD, and Riley J. Williams, III, MD

Because the 4-strand hamstring tendon graft is known to have a load to failure of over 4000 Newtons (N) and a strength that approximates that of a similarly sized patellar tendon graft,[1] the quadrupled hamstring tendon graft is an attractive choice for anterior cruciate ligament (ACL) reconstruction. Use of the hamstring autograft ACL reconstruction does not disturb the extensor mechanism of the knee, thus avoiding the potential morbidity associated with harvesting the patellar tendon. Proponents of bone-patellar tendon-bone autografts often state that they prefer the security of initial bone-to-bone fixation that is provided with the interference screw fixation typically used with these grafts. As such, the initial fixation strength of a hamstring ACL reconstruction has long been considered the weak link of this technique. Optimizing initial graft fixation in ACL reconstruction has been a focus for both surgeons and industry over the past 25 years. Consequently, the fixation strengths for devices used to secure soft-tissue ACL grafts have improved considerably. Currently, the authors recommend the use of a cross-pin fixation device for 4-strand hamstring tendon ACL grafts on the femoral side using the Bio-TransFix implant (Arthrex, Naples, FL), and the Intrafix device (Depuy-Mitek, Westwood, MA) for graft fixation on the tibial side (Figure 19-1).

There are 2 fixation types for ACL grafts in bone tunnels: aperture fixation and suspensory fixation. Aperture fixation describes graft fixation at the opening of the bone tunnel, typically with an interference screw. Suspensory fixation describes graft fixation that is remote from the intra-articular space (ie, at the femoral or tibial cortices). Suspensory fixation approaches include graft fixation using a screw (post) and washer, graft fixation using sutures suspended from a femoral fixation device such at the EndoButton (Smith & Nephew, Andover, MA), or graft fixation using a cross-pin type device (so-called cortico-cancellous fixation). The primary goal of initial fixation in ACL reconstruction is to resist graft slippage until tendon-to-bone healing occurs; ACL grafts should be stable

Figure 19-1. (A) Bio-TransFix femoral cross-pin soft-tissue graft-fixation device. (B) Intrafix sleeve-screw for fixation of soft-tissue grafts on the tibial side.

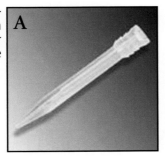
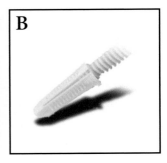

enough to withstand the physiologic loads applied to the knee during activities of daily living (ADLs). Moreover, graft fixation should also allow for the application of accelerated rehabilitation protocols. Ultimately, successful tendon to bone healing should occur without tunnel widening. The native ACL resists an estimated load of up to 454 N during activities of daily living.[2] The initial fixation of a soft-tissue graft should be able to resist this magnitude of load to be successful.

Femoral Fixation

For soft-tissue ACL grafts, both cortico-cancellous cross-pin fixation and cortical suspensory (eg, EndoButton) fixation have demonstrated superior graft stability and strength compared to aperture fixation (interference screws) on the femoral side in laboratory studies. In a study by Ahmad et al, the load-to-failure and graft slippage profile of the Bio-TransFix device was superior to that of the EndoButton CL, and an interference screw in porcine femora.[3] In this study, the Bio-TransFix cross-pin device (tendons pass over the pin within the femoral tunnel) was also superior to a cross-pin fixation device that pierced the tendon graft (Rigidfix, Mitek, Westwood, MA). Kousa et al compared the initial fixation strength of 6 femoral fixation devices for soft-tissue grafts in porcine femora.[4] These authors found that the Bone Mulch Screw (Arthrotek, Warsaw, IN), which is also a cross-pin fixation device, had a load to failure of 1112 N and had the lowest graft displacement (2.2 mm) when compared to the EndoButton CL (1086 N) and 3 interference screws (all less than 800 N load to failure).

The literature suggests that cross-pin fixation that does not pierce the ACL graft (eg, Bone Mulch Screw, TransFix, Bio-TransFix) are sufficiently strong enough to withstand knee forces associated with ADLs after ACL reconstruction. Both the cross-pin and suspensory techniques were consistently stronger when used with a soft-tissue graft compared to interference screw fixation on the femoral side. Some authors describe increased graft motion within the bony tunnels (bungee cord or windshield wiper effect) that is associated with the use of the EndoButton fixation device. The remote cortical fixation associated with the use of the EndoButton may correlate to the tunnel widening phenomena that is often observed after hamstring ACL reconstruction.[5] We prefer the Bio-TransFix device because it requires the drilling of a relatively short femoral tunnel compared to using the EndoButton. Use of the BioTransFix facilitates the application of strong early fixation that lies approximately 20 to 25 mm from the femoral tunnel opening.

Technique

After drilling the femoral tunnel to approximately 35 to 40 mm, a jig that includes an intra-articular hook and a lateral drill guide is seated in the tibial and femoral tunnels. A guide pin is drilled from lateral to medial in through both femoral cortices. The guide pin is pulled medially and replaced by a guide wire. This guide wire is pulled inferiorly out through the tibial tunnel. The ACL graft is loaded through the wire loop that has emerged from the tibial tunnel and pulled into the femoral tunnel by simultaneously pulling both ends of the wire. The Bio-TransFix device is then implanted into the distal femur (lateral to medial) over the wire and through the axilla of the ACL graft. The head of the implant should sit flush with the lateral femoral cortex (Figure 19-2).

Tibial Fixation

Because the tibial bone quality (density) is variable and often inferior to that of the femur, tibial fixation is considered more problematic compared to femoral fixation in hamstring ACL reconstruction.[6] Kousa et al compared 6 different tibial fixation devices in porcine tibiae, and found that the Intrafix device had the highest stiffness (223 N) and highest load to failure (1332 N).[6] This device utilizes a sleeve-screw configuration that allows for the tensioning of the individual graft limbs and maximizes apposition of the graft tendon ends to bone within the tunnel. The WasherLoc (Arthrotek, Warsaw, IN; 975 N) was also superior to a group of interference screws and a post/washer device in this study. Because the WasherLoc requires the removal of a large quantity of anteromedial tibial bone to seat the implant, we prefer the Intrafix to this device.

Technique

After fixing the graft on the femoral side, the graft is cycled to remove creep. With the knee slightly flexed (20 degrees), tension is put upon each of the four strands of the quadrupled tendon graft. A sheath trial (tap) is advanced into the tibial tunnel centrally between the limbs of each graft strand. The tap is removed and the Intrafix sheath is then impacted into the tibial tunnel until flush with the cortex. The IntraFix screw (typically size 8 to 10 mm) is advanced into the sleeve. Advancement of the screw causes expansion of the sleeve and compression of each tendon strand separately against the wall of the tibial tunnel (see Figure 19-2).

Clearly there are several different choices for graft fixation on both the femoral and tibial sides that can yield successful results following ACL reconstruction using a hamstring or soft-tissue graft. Biomechanical studies suggest that interference screw fixation alone for fixation of a hamstring graft is inferior to cross-pin fixation on the femoral side and second-generation fixation devices (Intrafix and WasherLoc) on the tibial side. Because these newer soft-tissue graft-fixation devices often require more steps for insertion compared to those steps needed to use the typical interference screw, we recommend performing these techniques in a cadaver or saw-bones model prior to using these implants in the operating room.

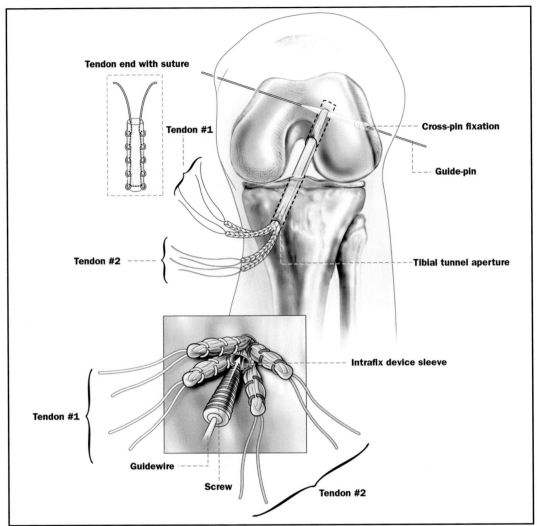

Figure 19-2. The authors' current method of femoral (cross-pin) and tibial (screw-sleeve) fixation for anterior cruciate ligament reconstruction with a hamstring tendon autograft. (Reprinted with permission from Williams RJ III, Hyman J, Petrigliano F, Rozental T, Wickiewicz TL. Anterior cruciate ligament reconstruction with a four-strand hamstring tendon autograft. Surgical technique. *J Bone Joint Surg Am.* 2005;87[suppl 1, pt 1]:51-66.)

References

1. Simonian PT, Williams RJ, Deng XH, Wickiewicz TL, Warren RF. Hamstring and patellar tendon graft response to cyclical loading. *Am J Knee Surg.* 1998;11(2):101-105.
2. Noyes FR, Butler DL, Grood ES, Zernicke RF, Hefzy MS. Biomechanical analysis of human ligament grafts used in knee-ligament repairs and reconstructions. *J Bone Joint Surg Am.* 1984;66(3):344-352.
3. Ahmad CS, Gardner TR, Groh M, Arnouk J, Levine WN. Mechanical properties of soft tissue femoral fixation devices for anterior cruciate ligament reconstruction. *Am J Sports Med.* 2004;32(3):635-640.
4. Kousa P, Jarvinen TL, Vihavainen M, Kannus P, Jarvinen M. The fixation strength of six hamstring tendon graft fixation devices in anterior cruciate ligament reconstruction. Part I: femoral site. *Am J Sports Med.* 2003; 31(2):174-181.

5. Williams RJ III, Hyman J, Petrigliano F, Rozental T, Wickiewicz TL. Anterior cruciate ligament reconstruction with a four-strand hamstring tendon autograft. *J Bone Joint Surg Am.* 2004;86-A(2):225-232.
6. Kousa P, Jarvinen TL, Vihavainen M, Kannus P, Jarvinen M. The fixation strength of six hamstring tendon graft fixation devices in anterior cruciate ligament reconstruction. Part II: tibial site. *Am J Sports Med.* 2003; 31(2):182-188.

How Do You Determine Tibial Tunnel Position to Optimize Graft Length and Femoral Tunnel Position When Performing an Endoscopic Technique?

Answorth A. Allen, MD

Graft-tunnel mismatch typically occurs during endoscopic anterior cruciate ligament (ACL) reconstruction when using a bone-patellar tendon-bone autograft or bone-patellar tendon-bone allograft. The basic problem is that if there is a graft tunnel mismatch, there will be an inadequate amount of bone in the tibial tunnel for interference screw fixation. It has been suggested that interference screw fixation cannot be done safely if there is less than 20 mm of bone in the tibial tunnel. However, in a porcine model, it has been shown that up to 12.5 mm of bone in the tibial tunnel maybe adequate for interference screw fixation. Several techniques have been developed to anticipate and to address the issue of graft-tunnel mismatch.[1-4]

Graft-tunnel mismatch typically occurs in patients whose patellar tendon length is equal to or greater than 50 mm. This does not necessarily correlate to the intra-articular distance between the femur and the tibia and the height of the patient. As the tibial tubercle guide angle is increased, the tibial tunnel becomes more vertical, and it gets increasingly more difficult to achieve anatomic placement of the femoral tunnel using standard endoscopic technique. A more vertical tibial tunnel can result in a femoral tunnel that is anterior and closer to the 12 o'clock position. The graft placement is then is non-anatomic and provides poor rotational control.

In 1993, Shaffer et al described a technique to anticipate and address graft tunnel mismatch.[1] They showed that the average length of the tibial tunnel (TT) necessary to achieve bitunnel fixation occurred when TT was equal to or greater than the length of the patellar tendon (LP) plus 20, minus the intra-articular distance (IAD): (TT $\geq$ LP + 20 − IAD). They were successful in predicting no graft-tunnel mismatch in 70% of the cases. In the other patients they addressed the graft-tunnel mismatch by recessing the graft in the femoral tunnel.

Hartman and Sisto described a technique where they measured the tibial tunnel length and intra-articular distance before committing to the femoral tunnel length.[2] Once the femoral tunnel length required to prevent a graft-tunnel mismatch was deduced, the femoral tunnel mismatch was then drilled. Their formula was TGL – (TTL + IAD), where TGL represents the total graft length and TTL represents the tibial tunnel length.

Miller et al described the N + 7 rule for tibial tunnel placement in endoscopic ACL reconstruction.[3] The tendinous portion of the graft is measured in millimeters and the number 7 is added to the graft length to determine the angle used for drilling the tibial tunnel. They created acceptable tunnels in 89% of their specimens. When using the N + 7 angle method the tibial guide is placed perpendicular to the axis of the tibia, the tunnel is started midway between the anterior tibial crest and the posteromedial corner of the tibia and exits through the posteromedial stump of the ACL. When using this technique, they were able to achieve bitunnel interference screw fixation in over 90% of the specimens. This is an indirect method of determining tibial tunnel length.

If there is graft-tunnel mismatch, there are several ways that are acceptable for addressing this clinically. One option is to consider an alternative fixation, such as using bioabsorbable screws. Another option is to create a bony trough at the outer aspect of the tibial tunnel, impacting the bone plug in the bony trough and fixing with 2 barbed staples. It has been shown by Gerich et al that staple fixation strength is equivalent to that of interference screw fixation.[4] Another technique involves flipping the tibial bone tunnel 180 degrees at the tendon insertion site, in essence effectively reducing the graft length. This will allow for stable fixation with an interference screw.

Others have recommended removal of a core of bone from the tibial tunnel and placing this on a soft-tissue portion of the graft in the tibial tunnel to allow for interference screw fixation.

Perhaps one of the simplest and most effective techniques to address graft-tunnel mismatch is rotation of the graft. Verma et al have shown that the graft can be rotated up to 540 degrees without compromising the strength of the graft.[5] This effectively shortened the graft up to 5.41 mm, representing approximately 10% of the effective length of the patellar tendon.

Author's Preferred Technique

In my opinion, the most important factor in ACL reconstruction is accurate tunnel placement. In primary cases, I prefer to use an endoscopic technique, but if there is a long patellar tendon (N > 50) with the potential for vertical tunnel placement, I will not hesitate to use alternative techniques such as a 2-incision technique, drilling the femoral tunnel through the medial portal or using a retro-guide. I prefer the N + 7 method to predict the angle of the guide. The tunnel is usually placed midway between the anterior tibial crest and the posteromedial corner, and I will try to exit in the anatomic center of the anterior cruciate ligament. From my clinical experience, the N + 7 rule prevents graft-tunnel mismatch in almost 95% of the cases, assuming that there is no intratendinous distance that is greater than 50 mm.

If there is graft-tunnel mismatch and this is less than 5 mm, my preferred technique is to rotate the graft and fix with a bioabsorbable screw. If the graft-tunnel mismatch is greater than 5 mm, then my preference is to create a trough in the proximal tibia and fix with 2 barbed staples.

References

1. Shaffer B, Gow W, Tibone JE. Graft-tunnel mismatch in endoscopic anterior cruciate ligament reconstruction: a new technique of intraarticular measurement and modified graft harvesting. *Arthroscopy.* 1993;9(6):633-646.
2. Hartman GP, Sisto DJ. Avoiding graft-tunnel mismatch in endoscopic anterior cruciate ligament reconstruction: a new technique. *Arthroscopy.* 1999;15(3):338-340.
3. Miller MD, Hinkin DR. The "N+7 rule" for tibial tunnel placement in endoscopic anterior cruciate ligament reconstruction. *Arthroscopy.* 1996;12:124-126.
4. Gerich JG, Cassim A, Lattermann C, Lobenhoffer HP. Pullout strength of tibial graft fixation in anterior cruciate ligament replacement with a patellar tendon graft: interference screw versus staple fixation in human knees. *Knee Surg Sports Trauamtol Arthrosc.* 1997;5(2):84-88.
5. Verma N, Noerdlinger MA, Hallab N, Bush-Joseph CA, Bach BR Jr. Effects of graft rotation on initial biomechanical failure characteristics of bone patellar tendon-bone construct. *Am J Sports Med.* 2003;31(5):708-713.

SECTION III

POSTOPERATIVE QUESTIONS

HOW DO YOU MANAGE THE ACL PATIENT FOLLOWING RECONSTRUCTION?

John-Paul H. Rue, MD, LCDR, MC, USN, and Brian J. Cole, MD, MBA

Early rehabilitation protocols following anterior cruciate ligament (ACL) reconstruction often involved immobilization of the extremity for more than 6 weeks. This was thought to allow time for the graft to heal and the inflammatory phase to pass.[1] Unfortunately, this immobilization had adverse effects on articular cartilage, ligaments, and other structures about the knee. In order to overcome many of the common complications present during the early evolution of ACL reconstruction, Shelbourne and Nitz described an accelerated rehabilitation program with emphasis on early return of full extension and full weight bearing as tolerated.[2] This accelerated protocol has been controversial, however, due to concerns that it may place increased forces on the ACL graft, leading to increased anterior laxity. This does not appear to be the case, as Beynnon et al demonstrated no significant difference in anterior laxity in a prospective, randomized double-blind study between groups treated with an accelerated or nonaccelerated ACL reconstruction protocol.[3] Our ACL rehabilitation protocol is based on the previously mentioned accelerated model because of the decreased likelihood of arthrofibrosis and other complications and improved strength and range of motion. In general, the accelerated ACL rehabilitation protocol described below encompasses many of the lessons learned from earlier, less aggressive protocols.[4]

Our primary rehabilitation goals following ACL reconstruction are progressive weight bearing, restoration of motion with emphasis on full extension, quadriceps strengthening, control of inflammation, and restoration of normal gait. In order to accomplish these goals, we often divide the rehabilitation program into phases,[5] with each phase getting progressively more complex (Figure 21-1).

Phase 1 is from 0 to 4 weeks postoperative. During this time, patients are weight bearing as tolerated with crutches. They are placed in a range-of-motion brace locked in full extension for ambulation and sleeping for the first week. From weeks 1 to 4, the brace

	WEIGHT BEARING	BRACE	ROM	THERAPEUTIC EXERCISES
PHASE I **0 - 4 weeks**	As tolerated with crutches*	**0-1 week**: locked in full extension for ambulation and sleeping **1-4 weeks**: unlocked for ambulation, remove for sleeping**	As tolerated	Heel slides, quad/hamstring sets, patellar mobs, gastroc/soleus stretch***, SLR with brace in full extension until quad strength prevents extension lag
PHASE II **4 - 6 weeks**	Gradually discontinue crutch use	Discontinue use when patient has full extension and no extension lag	Maintain full extension and progressive flexion	Progress to weight bearing gastroc/soleus stretch, begin toe raises, closed chain extension, balance exercises, hamstring curls, and stationary bike
PHASE III **6 weeks - 4 months**	Full, without use of crutches and with a normalized gait pattern	None	Gain full and pain-free	Advance closed chain strengthening, progress proprioception activities, begin Stairmaster/Nordic Trac and running straight ahead at 12 weeks
PHASE IV **4 - 6 months**	Full	None	Full and pain-free	Progress flexibility/strengthening, progression of function: forward/ backward running, cutting, grapevine, etc., initiate plyometric program and sport-specific drills
PHASE V **6 months and beyond**	Full	None	Full and pain-free	Gradual return to sports participation, maintenance program for strength and endurance

*Modified with concomitantly performed meniscus repair/transplantation or articular cartilage procedure
**Brace may be removed for sleeping after first post-operative visit (day 7-10)
***This exercise is to be completed in a non-weight bearing position

Figure 21-1. Anterior cruciate ligament reconstruction rehabilitation phases. (ROM = range of motion; SLR = straight leg raises) (Reprinted from Cole B. ACL patellar tendon allograft/autograft reconstruction rehabilitation program. Available at: http://www.cartilagedoc.org. Accessed October 1, 2006.)

is unlocked for ambulation and removed for sleeping. Their range of motion is as tolerated. The therapist will specifically work with them on prone leg hangs (Figure 21-2), heel slides, quadriceps and hamstring sets, patellar mobility, gastrocnemius and soleus stretching, and straight leg raises with brace in full extension until quadriceps function returns and there is no longer an extension lag.

Phase 2 is from 4 to 6 weeks. During this time, patients will gradually discontinue the use of crutches. The brace may be discontinued when full extension has been achieved and the patient no longer has an extension lag. The goals for motion are to maintain full extension and progress with flexion as tolerated. The therapist will specifically work with them on progressing to weight-bearing gastrocnemius and soleus stretching, beginning toe raises, closed-chain extension, balance exercises, hamstring curls, and riding a stationary bike.

Phase 3 is from 6 weeks to 4 months. This is the longest phase because it primarily focuses on progressing quadriceps and hamstring strengthening. Patients should have a normal gait without the use of crutches or a brace. Range of motion should be full and pain free. The therapist will specifically work with patients on advanced closed-chain strengthening, progressive proprioception activities, initiating cross-training exercises, and running straight ahead beginning at 12 weeks.

Phase 4 is from 4 to 6 months. Patients progress with flexibility and strengthening and begin progression of function exercises such as running backwards and cutting and pivoting. Plyometric exercise programs and sport-specific drills are initiated.

Phase 5 is from 6 months and beyond. Gradual return to sports participation is allowed and patients continue with a maintenance program for strength and endurance.

Disclaimer

The views expressed in this article are those of the author and do not necessarily reflect the official policy or position of the Department of the Navy, Department of Defense, nor the United States Government.

References

1. Paulos L, Noyes F, Grood E, Butler D. Knee rehabilitation after anterior cruciate ligament reconstruction and repair. *Am J Sports Med.* 1981;9:140-149.
2. Shelbourne K, Nitz P. Accelated rehabilitation after anterior cruciate ligament reconstruction. *Am J Sports Med.* 1990;18:292-299.
3. Beynnon B, Uh B, Johnson R, et al. Open versus closed kinetic chain exercises in patellofemoral pain: a 5-year prospective randomized study. *Am J Sports Med.* 2005;33:347-359.
4. Wilk K, Reinold M, Hooks T. Recent advances in the rehabilitation of isolated and combined anterior cruciate ligament injuries. *Orthop Clin N Am.* 2003;34:107-137.
5. Cole B. ACL patellar tendon allograft/autograft reconstruction rehabilitation program. Available at: http://www.cartilagedoc.org. Accessed October 1, 2006.

DO YOU REHAB YOUR PATELLAR TENDON AUTOGRAFT AND ALLOGRAFT PATIENTS DIFFERENTLY?

John-Paul H. Rue, MD, LCDR, MC, USN, and Brian J. Cole, MD, MBA

No, the rehabilitation is the same regardless of whether I use patellar tendon autograft or allograft. Many of my patients report less pain initially with allograft reconstruction, but this usually resolves within the first few weeks and after that there is no appreciable difference between the 2 graft sources. This has been validated by several authors who have reported no significant difference in long-term outcomes between anterior cruciate ligament (ACL) reconstructions with patellar tendon autografts and allografts using similar accelerated rehabilitation protocols.[1,2]

The current sterilization techniques for bone-patellar tendon-bone (BTB) allograft tissue are aseptic harvesting, cryopreservation, and gamma radiation with low-dose radiation of less than 3.0 Mrad.[3] These techniques have been shown to be the most effective methods of producing a sterile ACL graft and maximizing structural integrity while minimizing disease transmission and are significant improvements over previous methods of sterilization, which often compromised the structural integrity of the allografts.[4]

The initial graft tensile strength of BTB autograft is 2977 N (Newtons) with a stiffness of 620 N/mm.[5] The strength and stiffness are similar for BTB autografts and allografts that have been sterilized using the previously mentioned techniques.[6] We use interference screws for both the femoral and tibial fixation in a similar fashion for both graft choices. This fixation provides bone-to-bone healing in approximately 6 weeks for autografts. Longer bone-to-bone healing rates of greater than 6 months have been reported due to slower incorporation in allografts.[6,7] There is no evidence that this delay in bone-to-bone healing has any detrimental effect on the strength of the allograft reconstruction.

Both autograft and allograft tissues (Figures 22-1 and 22-2) undergo a process of ligamentization, and both initially decrease in strength and then subsequently undergo gradual increases in strength. This entire revascularization process typically occurs over a 5-month period. By 6 months, both grafts resemble normally oriented connective tissue,

Figure 22-1. BTB autograft.

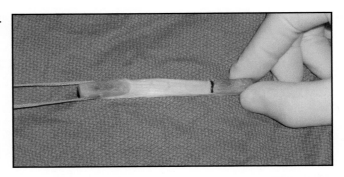

Figure 22-2. BTB allograft.

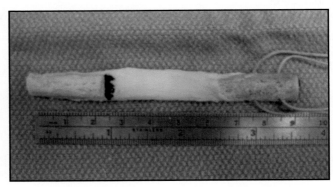

and histological studies have shown no difference in allograft and autograft BTB grafts at 1 year.[8] Because allograft and autograft BTB grafts are similar in their structural and mechanical properties, we believe it is reasonable to follow the same postoperative rehabilitation protocols for either graft choice.[9]

My rehabilitation protocol is focused on achieving several goals. These are progressive weight bearing, restoration of motion with emphasis on full extension, quadriceps strengthening, control of inflammation, and restoration of normal gait. Because the grafts are similar in their structural and mechanical properties (Table 22-1), the goals of rehabilitation and how we achieve them are the same regardless of whether the patient has a BTB allograft or autograft. As mentioned previously, many of my patients who have allograft ACL reconstructions may experience less pain than their autograft counterparts. In fact, a subset of this population may attempt to exceed the biologic properties of the allograft because of the minimum amount of pain that they experience. I have found that when properly educated about these time-dependent properties, these patients will slow down their rehabilitation accordingly.

Disclaimer

The views expressed in this article are those of the author and do not necessarily reflect the official policy or position of the Department of the Navy, Department of Defense, nor the United States Government.

Table 22-1
Comparison of Bone-Patellar Tendon-Bone Autograft and Allograft

Graft	Bone-to-Bone Fixation?	Timing of Bone-to-Bone Healing	Duration of Revascularization and Ligamentization
Bone-patellar tendon-bone autograft	Yes	6 to 10 weeks	5 to 6 months
Bone-patellar tendon-bone allograft	Yes	Up to 1 year	5 to 6 months

References

1. Harner C, Olson E, Irrgang J, Silverstein S, Fu F, Silbey M. Allograft versus autograft anterior cruciate ligament reconstruction: 3- to 5-year outcome. *Clin Orthop Relat Res.* 1996;324:134-144.
2. Shelton W, Papendick L, Dukes A. Autograft versus allograft anterior cruciate ligament reconstruction. *Arthroscopy.* 1997;13:446-449.
3. West R, Harner C. Graft selection in anterior cruciate ligament reconstruction. *J Am Acad Orthop Surg.* 2005; 13:197-207.
4. Vangsness C, Garcia I, Mills C, Kainer M, Roberts M, Moore T. Allograft transplantation in the knee: tissue regulation, procurement, processing, and sterilization. *Am J Sports Med.* 2003;31:474-481.
5. Noyes F, Butler D, Grood E, Zernicke R, Hefzy M. Biomechanical analysis of human ligament grafts used in knee-ligament repairs and reconstructions. *J Bone Joint Surg Am.* 1984;66:344-352.
6. Markholf K, Burchfield D, Shapiro M, Cha C, Finerman G, Slauterbeck J. Biomechanical consequences of replacement of the anterior cruciate ligament with a patellar ligament allograft: II. Forces in the graft compated with forces in the intact ligament. *J Bone Joint Surg Am.* 1996;78:1728-1734.
7. Arnoczky S. Biology of ACL reconstructions. What happens to the graft? *Instr Course Lect.* 1996;45:229-233.
8. Arnoczky S, Warren R, Ashlock M. Replacement of the anterior cruciate ligament using a patellar tendon allograft. An experimental study. *J Bone Joint Surg Am.* 1986;68:376-385.
9. Cole B. ACL patellar tendon allograft/autograft reconstruction rehabilitation program. Available at: http://www.cartilagedoc.org. Accessed October 1, 2006.

Do You Manage the Patient Differently if a Concurrent Meniscal Repair Was Performed?

John-Paul H. Rue, MD, LCDR, MC, USN, and Brian J. Cole, MD, MBA

Numerous studies have reported improved healing rates for meniscal repairs when performed concurrently with anterior cruciate ligament (ACL) reconstruction (Table 23-1). Barber and Click demonstrated in 1997 that patients undergoing simultaneous ACL reconstruction with meniscal repair had a 92% healing rate in ACL-reconstructed knees, versus 67% in ACL-deficient knees.[1] There are several possible explanations for this, including a blood-filled joint and the elimination of joint instability, all of which lead to a more favorable healing environment for the meniscal repair.[2]

Other than a minor alteration in weight-bearing status, there is no difference in our rehabilitation for an ACL reconstruction with concomitant meniscal repair compared to that done for an ACL reconstruction performed in isolation.[3] We allow our patients who have simultaneous ACL reconstruction and meniscal repairs to be weight bearing as tolerated in extension. We do not allow any weight bearing in flexion of 90 degrees or more for 4 weeks. After 4 weeks, progressive weight bearing in flexion is allowed.

The rationale for this restriction of weight bearing in higher degrees of flexion is supported by work by Thompson et al, who demonstrated 5.1 mm of posterior displacement of the medial meniscus with flexion and 11.2 mm of displacement for the lateral meniscus. Numerous causes for meniscal repair failure have been hypothesized. However, the most predictable measures of repair success are tear pattern and vascularity at the site of the meniscal tear, with longitudinal tears in the red-red zone having the highest rates of healing.[6] A recent study showed that loads across a lateral meniscal repair are compressive throughout flexion and extension, with the highest loads measured in full extension and the lowest loads at 90 degrees of flexion.[4] Our belief is that this amount of displacement may cause significant shearing at the repair site and contribute to failure of the meniscal repair.

Table 23-1
Results of Meniscal Repair Performed in Conjunction With Anterior Cruciate Ligament Reconstruction

Author and Year	Number of Meniscal Repairs	Mean Follow-Up (Months)	Results
Tenuta and Arciero, 1994[5]	40	11	90% Healed
Buseck and Noyes, 1991[6]	79	12	80% Healed completely 14% Healed partially
Miller, 1988[7]	60	39	93% Healed

Many orthopedic surgeons do not change their rehabilitation protocols for their patients with concomitant meniscal repairs, following the ACL protocol as usual, and have reported no significant adverse outcomes and comparable meniscal repair healing rates.[6,8-10]

Disclaimer

The views expressed in this article are those of the author and do not necessarily reflect the official policy or position of the Department of the Navy, Department of Defense, nor the United States Government.

References

1. Barber F, Click S. Meniscus repair rehabilitation with concurrent anterior cruciate ligament reconstruction. *Arthroscopy*. 1997;13:433-437.
2. Kimura M, Shirakura K, Haseqawa A, Kobuna Y, Niijima M. Second look arthroscopy after meniscal repair. Factors affecting the healing rate. *Clin Orthop Relat Res*. 1995;314:185-191.
3. Dehaven K, Arnoczky S. Meniscus repair: basic science, indications for repair, and open repair. *Instr Course Lect*. 1994;43:65-76.
4. Richards D, Barber F, Herbert M. Compressive loads in longitudinal lateral meniscus tears: a biomechanical study in porcine knees. *Arthroscopy*. 2005;21:1452-1456.
5. Tenuta J, Arciero R. Arthroscopic evaluation of meniscal repairs: factors that effect healing. *Am J Sports Med*. 1994;22(6):797-802.
6. Buseck M, Noyes F. Arthroscopic evaluation of meniscal repairs after anterior cruciate ligament reconstruction and immediate motion. *Am J Sports Med*. 1991;19:489-494.
7. Miller D Jr. Arthroscopic meniscus repair. *Am J Sports Med*. 1988;16:315-320.
8. Bach B, Levy M, Bojchuk J, Tradonsky S, Bush-Joseph C, Khan N. Single-incision endoscopic anterior cruciate ligament reconstruction using patellar tendon autograft. Minimum two-year follow-up evaluation. *Am J Sports Med*. 1998;26:30-40.
9. Barber F. Accelerated rehabilitation for meniscus repairs. *Arthroscopy*. 1994;10:206-210.
10. Greis P, Holmstrom M, Bardana D, Burks R. Meniscal injury: II. Management. *J Am Acad Orthop Surg*. 2002;10:177-187.

How Do You Manage the Patient Who Is Having a Difficult Time Gaining Extension After Reconstruction?

Eric C. McCarty, MD, and Brian Kerr, MD

Loss of motion, particularly extension, following anterior cruciate ligament (ACL) reconstruction presents a serious problem with potentially significant deleterious effects on patient outcomes. A loss of 3 to 5 degrees of extension compared to the opposite knee can result in lower postoperative objective scores.[1] We find that patients with less extension in one knee protect that knee, and over time the stiff knee becomes weaker. Loss of extension is usually more problematic than loss of flexion.[2]

Obviously, the best way to treat this problem is to take purposeful steps to prevent the potential for postoperative extension loss both before surgery and intraoperatively. We have a strict preoperative ACL reconstruction protocol that emphasizes, among other goals, extension to at least 0 degrees before surgery is undertaken.[3] This involves allowing time for the acute knee effusion to resolve and for specific range of motion exercises aimed at restoring full extension. Sufficient ACL remnant debridement and accurate tunnel placement—along with visualization of the ACL graft with the knee in full extension—during surgery help to ensure that there will be no physical block to obtaining full motion.

Despite strict adherence to the above principles, extension loss can still occur. We like to monitor our patients' rehabilitation closely in the first weeks after surgery to quickly identify any patients who develop difficulty in regaining extension. If we find patients whose extension is falling behind early in the postoperative period (during the first 3 weeks), we point out the problem to them, emphasize the importance of regaining their extension, and encourage a renewed dedication to their extension exercises. We repeat instructions for our protocol emphasizing extension-based exercises and remind them to help prevent worsening of the problem by refraining from such practices as placing a pillow behind the knee for comfort. Instead, we encourage them to place a pillow or other prop under the heel while sitting to allow the knee to fall into full extension. Specific exercises are again prescribed, such as prone hangs and towel stretches, in which the patient

Figure 24-1. Towel stretches. One hand holds firm pressure on the thigh while the other hand pulls the foot off the table, fully extending the knee.

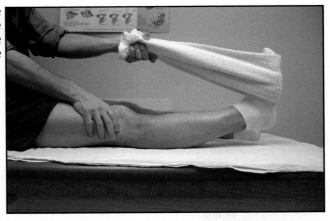

Figure 24-2. Knee with flexion contracture placed in extension board.

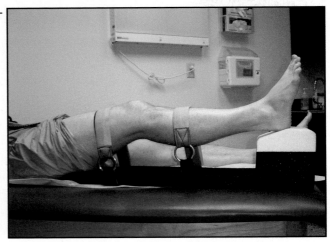

is sitting with the leg extended with one hand holding a towel that is looped around the arch of the foot and the other hand holding downward pressure on the thigh. The towel is then pulled, with the goal of pulling the foot off of the table, eventually pulling the knee into hyperextension (Figure 24-1).

When extension deficits persist or develop longer than one month postoperatively, more aggressive and focused treatment is required. An extension board is a simple and effective tool in overcoming extension deficits (Full Extension Knee Device, Lansing, MI). The patient's heel is place on a raised padded platform, and straps are placed under tension over the thigh and leg (Figure 24-2). Over time, the knee is eventually stretched to full or hyperextension (Figure 24-3). Our formula for most patients is "3 × 10 = 0", meaning 3 sessions of extension board use per day, for 10 minutes per session, will produce extension to 0 degress. There are many commercially available extension boards, from very simple to more sophisticated models in which the patient can continually adjust tension while lying supine.

For patients who fail to respond quickly to extension board use, or who prove noncompliant to the prescribed schedule of usage, we recommend extension casting. A well-padded fiberglass cast is applied to the knee in the maximum degree of extension that

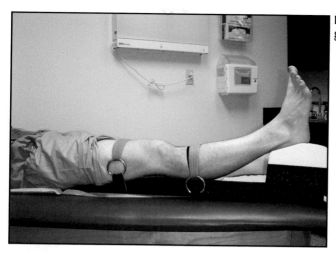

Figure 24-3. Resulting extension gain after use of extension board.

can be tolerated by the patient. This can be fashioned with a dropout back to allow for range-of-motion exercises.

When aggressive stretching fails to yield further improvements beyond 12 to 16 weeks, we recommend arthroscopic scar resection for the resultant arthrofibrosis. An initial manipulation under anesthesia is performed, with the resultant range of motion noted. The first and most common intra-articular scar site to be addressed is the bulbous cyclops lesion at the anterior base of the ACL graft. This is resected until the knee can be brought into full extension without impingement. If adequate cyclops resection fails to allow full extension, further arthroscopic scar debridement is undertaken, particularly tissue near the anterior fat pad anterior to the horns of the medial and lateral menisci. Parapatellar scar tissue can also be released medially and laterally in the suprapatellar pouch.[2] Additionally, further notchplasty can be undertaken if bony impingement is noted along the ACL graft. Finally, an additional knee manipulation is performed following scar release to obtain full flexion and extension. A fiberglass cast can then be applied with the knee in full extension, again with the option for a dropout back.

Postoperatively, an immediate aggressive program is followed utilizing many of the previously mentioned stretches and exercises, reapplying the extension cast for overnight use if necessary.

Prevention of factors leading to extension loss remains our best defense against postoperative stiffness. However, once extension loss does occur, we prefer an aggressive approach to treating the condition, with emphasis to the patient on the importance of focused attention and effort in combating the problem.

References

1. Shelbourne KD, Klotz C. What I have learned about the ACL: utilizing a progressive rehabilitation scheme to achieve total knee symmetry after ACL reconstruction. *J Orthop Sci*. 2006;11(3):318-325.
2. Shelbourne KD, Patel DV. Classification and management of arthrofibrosis of the knee after ACL reconstruction. *Am J Sports Med*. 1996;24:857-862.
3. Multicenter Orthopaedic Outcomes Network. *Perioperative Anterior Cruciate Ligament Reconstruction Protocol*. Nashville, TN: 2007.

HOW DO YOU MANAGE THE PATIENT WHO DEVELOPS A POSTOPERATIVE INFECTION FOLLOWING ACL RECONSTRUCTION?

Matthew T. Provencher, MD, LCDR, MC, USN, and Nikhil N. Verma, MD

Infections following anterior cruciate ligament (ACL) reconstruction are infrequent, with an estimated incidence of less than 0.1% to 1%.[1-8] Even though septic arthritis after ACL reconstruction is uncommon, the infection may have serious consequences. Postsurgical infections can be classified based on temporal course after the surgery as well as presumed location of infection (Table 25-1). A patient who presents with concerns of a postsurgical infection should have his history reviewed to ensure that he does not have additional risk factors that may predispose to infection, such as immunosuppression, cancer history, or prior irradiation to the knee. Additionally, he should be questioned regarding new onset of malaise, general fatigue, increasing discomfort in the knee rather than gradual improvement, increasing or persistent drainage from surgical incisions, night sweats, and other symptoms associated with generalized infection.

A thorough physical examination should include vitals and assessment of infectious signs such as prominent or painful proximal lymph nodes (femoral/inguinal) and lymphedema or lymph streaking. The knee examination should first start with inspection to assess for swelling and/or effusion, presence of erythema (diffuse or streaking), and any persistent wound drainage of patient dressings. An assessment of passive knee range-of-motion pain should be complete while the knee is gently flexed and extended to signify inflammation of the knee synovial lining suggestive of infection. Wounds should be gently probed superficially with a sterile cotton tip applicator to assess communication with deeper structures.

If there is an effusion, our approach is to perform a diagnostic aspiration from a peripatellar lateral approach, away from any prior incisions, by gently tilting the patella laterally and inserting an 18-gauge to 20-gauge needle with a 20-cc syringe. Any fluid

Table 25-1

Classification of Postoperative Septic Arthritis, Based on Temporal Course and Location of Infection

Postsurgical Timing[2,4,5,7]	*Acute (<2 weeks)*	*Subacute (2 to 8 weeks)*	*Late (>2 months)*
Location of infection	Superficial; wound dehiscence, stitch abscess	Intra-articular; joint fluid, capsule	Intraosseous; osteo-myelitis

Table 25-2

Diagnostic Criteria to Suggest Postoperative Septic Arthritis

Usually Present	*Sometimes Present*	*Rarely Present*
Persistent drainage from incisions, especially tibial wound	Pain with passive knee range of motion[2,6-8]	Severe pain[2]
Persistent effusion or swelling and warmth	Local or streaking erythema, possible lymphadenopathy	Chills or systemic symptoms[2]
Increased difficulty performing physical therapy[7]	Systemic signs, fever[5,7]	Blood cultures rarely positive[7]
Joint fluid aspirate white cell count usually elevated (greater than 10 to 15K, but usually 30 to 50K minimum)	Elevated peripheral WBC count	
Granulocyte or PMN count of >90% in joint fluid		
Elevated ESR and CRP		

PMN = polymorphonuclear leukocytes; ESR = erythrocyte sedimentation rate; CRP = C-reactive protein; WBC = white blood count

obtained should be sent for immediate cell count and Gram stain analysis and be processed for culture. The gold standard to diagnose a knee infection remains fluid or tissue culture. The culture results may be falsely negative in the setting of prior oral or parenteral antibiotic administration. It should be noted that postoperative septic arthritis, especially after ACL reconstruction, might be present despite a relatively benign patient presentation. It is incumbent upon the surgeon to perform a thorough workup, including examination, peripheral blood counts (complete blood count [CBC], erythrocyte sedimentation rate [ESR], and C-reactive protein [CRP]), and joint aspiration if indicated to rule out infection (Table 25-2).

The CRP and ESR may be important markers for postoperative septic arthritis, even though it is known that both of these values may be elevated after surgery.[9] It has been shown,[9] however, that there is a predictable decline in both ESR and CRP after a peak between the third and seventh day after ACL reconstruction; however, the CRP consistently demonstrates a more rapid return to normal. Thus, CRP may be used as a more accurate predictor that ESR for postoperative septic arthritis given a clinical picture consistent with infection. CRP may be good laboratory marker to assess improvement.

It is not required to have a confirmed diagnosis of postoperative ACL infection prior to surgical intervention. In light of a presumed infection, with sufficient clinical and historical evidence to suggest, the surgeon may offer the patient the option of proceeding to operative intervention without aspiration or waiting for culture results. It should be assumed that any patient who requires operative intervention after ACL reconstruction should undergo a thorough lavage and intra-articular debridement with the optimal goal of preserving the reconstructed ACL tissue. The goals of treatment for a patient with septic arthritis after ACL reconstructions are to not only protecting the ACL graft but also the articular cartilage.[5]

Early and prompt recognition, followed by arthroscopic lavage and debridement, may allow the ACL graft to be saved[2,4,5,7,8] and help to limit articular cartilage damage.[5] However, all suspicious areas of infection around the knee should be addressed, including the tibial wound, and in cases of bone-tendon-bone (BTB) reconstruction, the patellar wound. We feel that arthroscopic lavage and debridement can safely eradicate the infection with less morbidity of an open arthrotomy. Sequential arthroscopic lavage should be considered, with several operations over the course of 7 to 10 days.[2,4,5,7,8] The ACL graft status should be documented; however, we feel it should be left alone in the initial debridement. If the infection is persistent and remains unresponsive to serial debridements and IV antibiotics, then graft and hardware removal should be considered.[4,5,7,8] It is recommended that postoperative drains be utilized for 2 to 4 days.[4,5,7,8]

Parenteral postoperative antibiotics should be given in scheduled doses, with a broad-spectrum antibiotic (Cefazolin or equivalent). Final antibiotic choice and dosage should be adjusted once final cultures are available. In areas of high methicillin-resistant organisms, additional antibiotics should be given prior to receiving the final culture results.

The overall characteristics and results of patients treated for septic arthritis after ACL reconstructions are summarized. Since few infections are reported, there is continued debate regarding the optimal management of postoperative septic arthritis. In a survey of 61 surgeons, Matava[6] reported 5 different methods to treat surgical infection and recommended that if the ACL graft was removed, revision surgery should not be considered before 6 to 9 months. Our current treatment recommendations are in line with the results of Matava's[6] survey: once an infection is encountered, IV antibiotics (culture-specific) and irrigation/lavage with graft retention as the initial treatment; in cases of resistant infections, graft and hardware removal is necessary, with consideration of revision surgery in approximately 6 months. With prompt recognition and surgical treatment, the potential complications of septic arthritis such as arthrofibrosis, chondral damage, graft damage, and bone tunnel enlargement may be minimized or avoided.

References

1. Babcock HM, Carroll C, Matava M, L'Ecuyer P, Fraser V. Surgical site infections after arthroscopy: Outbreak investigation and case control study. *Arthroscopy*. 2003;19(2):172-181.

2. Burks RT, Friederichs MG, Fink B, Luker MG, West HS, Greis PE. Treatment of postoperative anterior cruciate ligament infections with graft removal and early reimplantation. *Am J Sports Med.* 2003;31(3):414-418.
3. Crawford C, Kainer M, Jernigan D, et al. Investigation of postoperative allograft-associated infections in patients who underwent musculoskeletal allograft implantation. *Clin Infect Dis.* 2005;41(2):195-200.
4. Fong SY, Tan JL. Septic arthritis after arthroscopic anterior cruciate ligament reconstruction. *Ann Acad Med Singapore.* 2004;33(2):228-234.
5. Indelli PF, Dillingham M, Fanton G, Schurman DJ. Septic arthritis in postoperative anterior cruciate ligament reconstruction. *Clin Orthop Relat Res.* 2002;398:182-188.
6. Margheritini F, Camillieri G, Mancini L, Mariani PP. C-reactive protein and erythrocyte sedimentation rate changes following arthroscopically assisted anterior cruciate ligament reconstruction. *Knee Surg Sports Traumatol Arthrosc.* 2001;9(6):343-345.
7. Matava MJ, Evans TA, Wright RW, Shively RA. Septic arthritis of the knee following anterior cruciate ligament reconstruction: results of a survey of sports medicine fellowship directors. *Arthroscopy.* 1998;14(7):717-725.
8. McAllister DR, Parker RD, Cooper AE, Recht MP, Abate J. Outcomes of postoperative septic arthritis after anterior cruciate ligament reconstruction. *Am J Sports Med.* 1999;27(5):562-570.
9. Williams RJ III, Laurencin CT, Warren RF, Speciale AC, Brause BD, O'Brien S. Septic arthritis after arthroscopic anterior cruciate ligament reconstruction. Diagnosis and management. *Am J Sports Med.* 1997;25(2):261-267.

How Do You Manage the Patient Who Has Postoperative Patellar Pain?

James D. Ferrari, MD

Patellar pain after anterior cruciate ligament (ACL) reconstruction is a common complaint among patients. It can range from mild annoyance when kneeling to severe interference with athletics and even activities of daily living. Clearly its occurrence after reconstruction is well recognized, but its cause remains somewhat enigmatic.

Sachs and colleagues noted an association of anterior knee pain with quadriceps weakness and postoperative flexion contracture.[1] Aglietti et al were able to significantly reduce the incidence of postoperative patellar problems by focusing on early motion with full extension.[2] Clearly it has been shown that obtaining early full hyperextension is the best prevention.[3] Nonetheless, donor site issues are a concern as well. Fewer problems with kneeling are seen in patients with hamstring autografts versus patellar tendon autografts.[4] Controversy exists as to whether kneeling pain after patellar tendon harvest is secondary to the graft being taken or the loss of sensation on the front of the knee. Preservation of the infrapatellar branches of the saphenous nerve during bone-patellar tendon-bone (BTB) graft harvesting has been shown to be critical in the patients' ability to kneel without pain.[5]

There is no doubt that obtaining full hyperextension after ACL reconstruction is the best prevention for postoperative patellar pain. What does one do when patellar pain is an issue, however? I look to have full hyperextension at the first postoperative visit. If this is not the case, have your patient do prone heel hangs with and without weights and consider using an extension board. If a large effusion is present at the first visit and quadriceps activity is poor, aspirate the knee. Have both the patient and the therapist work on improving patellofemoral mobility with manual manipulation and tissue massage in the suprapatellar pouch and medial and lateral gutters. Whether using patellar tendon grafts or hamstring tendons, scar tissue will form around the patellar tendon, tethering patellofemoral mobility. This usually peaks around 6 weeks postop. Deep tissue massage to the front of the knee helps loosen the tissue. Patients with thickened, inflamed soft tissues often benefit from a methylprednisolone dose pack, but wait until roughly 6 weeks postop to prescribe this.

Pain that persists despite these efforts often benefits from modalities such as ultrasound and cortisone iontophoresis. Although there is little data in the literature to support its use, I have had good experience in a few cases with extracorporeal shock wave lithotripsy. It is best used in recalcitrant cases in patients with good range of motion but isolated anterior knee pain or patellar tendonitis.

Severe cases of patellofemoral pain after ACL reconstruction associated with loss of flexion and/or extension often require operative intervention. Small losses of extension are more easily treated than larger losses of extension and flexion. Most small extension loss is secondary to a fibroproliferative nodule, the cyclops lesion. Patients will have a slight loss of hyperextension or a rubbery endpoint to full extension and will complain of retropatellar pain with extension and often a feeling of giving way with extension. Arthroscopic debridement of the cyclops lesion restores full extension and eliminates the quadriceps inhibition.

Larger losses of extension may require further debridement of intercondylar notch scarring. If the patellofemoral joint motion is severely inhibited, perform arthroscopic lateral and possibly even medial releases in order to restore patellar mobility. This will also help improve flexion loss. Occasionally a normal appearing, asymptomatic medial plica will become fibrotic and symptomatic after ACL reconstruction. Arthroscopic resection is sometimes necessary for complete resolution of pain.

Overall patellar pain after ACL reconstruction is secondary to loss of full extension, tethering of the patella secondary to scar tissue, and poor quadriceps strength. Rehab efforts directed at attaining full hyperextension, patellar mobility, and quad strength are of paramount importance. If despite these efforts patellar pain persists and the patient is unable to attain full hyperextension, consider operative means in order to restore full motion and normal patellofemoral mobility.

References

1. Sachs RA, Daniel DM, Stone ML, Garfein RF. Patellofemoral problems after anterior cruciate ligament reconstruction. *Am J Sports Med.* 1989;17:760-765.
2. Aglietti P, Buzzi R, D'Andria S, Zaccherotti G. Patellofemoral problems after intra-articular anterior cruciate ligament reconstruction. *Clin Orthop Rel Res.* 1993;288:195-204.
3. Shelbourne KD, Trumper RV. Preventing anterior knee pain after anterior cruciate ligament reconstruction. *Am J Sports Med.* 1997;25:41-47.
4. Spindler KP, Kuhn JE, Freedman KB, et al. Anterior cruciate ligament reconstruction autograft choice: bone-tendon-bone versus hamstring. *Am J Sport Med.* 2004;32:1986-1995.
5. Kartus J, Movin T, Karlsson J. Donor-site morbidity and anterior knee problems after anterior cruciate ligament reconstruction using autografts. *Arthroscopy.* 2001;17: 971-980.

How Do You Determine the Timing of Reoperation in a Patient Who Has Motion Problems Following an ACL Reconstruction?

James D. Ferrari, MD

Motion loss and arthrofibrosis of the knee following anterior cruciate ligament (ACL) reconstruction is oftentimes more debilitating than the initial injury and subsequent symptoms that precipitated the surgery itself. Historically, motion problems following ACL reconstruction in isolated ACL injuries range from as low as 2% to upwards of 25%.[1,2] Fortunately, a greater understanding of risk factors associated with arthrofibrosis, precise surgical technique, and early aggressive rehabilitation has decreased the incidence of motion problems.

Arthrofibrosis can be broadly categorized into three main types. The most commonly encountered type is localized arthrofibrosis, also known as the *cyclops lesion*. A localized nodule of fibroproliferative scar tissue attaches to the tibial side of the ACL graft, resulting in a mechanical block to full extension. Flexion is not affected. Infrapatellar contracture syndrome is caused by fibrosis of the fat pad, resulting in inferior translation of the patella, diminished patellofemoral mobility, and loss of both flexion and extension. Global arthrofibrosis is secondary to scarring and fibrosis of the medial and lateral gutters as well as the suprapatellar pouch and results in loss of both flexion and extension. In general, losses of flexion are much better tolerated than losses of extension. Even a few degrees of extension loss can lead to anterior knee pain, patellar tendonitis, and patellar cartilage overload.

Shelbourne and colleagues developed a 4-part classification scheme that is both descriptive and prognostic (Table 27-1).[3] Patients with type 4 severe arthrofibrosis fare the worst after surgical intervention, but gains are seen nonetheless.

Table 27-1

Classification Scheme for Arthrofibrosis

Type	Flexion Loss (degrees)	Extension Loss (degrees)
1	Normal	<10
2	Normal	>10
3	>25	>10
4	>30	>10 with patella infera

Adapted from Shelbourne KD, Patel DV, Martini DJ. Classification and management of arthrofibrosis of the knee after anterior cruciate ligament reconstruction. *Am J Sports Med.* 1996;24:857-862.

Timing of surgery to regain motion is dictated by the underlying cause of the motion loss. Losses of flexion and/or extension are numerous and multifactorial. Loss of extension can be secondary to notch impingement from a malpositioned graft, a cyclops lesion,[4] or inadequate notchplasty. Other causes include infrapatellar contracture syndrome, complex regional pain syndrome (CRPS), hamstring tightness, posterior capsular scarring, a tightened capsule from meniscal repair, or medial collateral ligament scarring. Causes of loss of flexion include improper graft position, suprapatellar and medial and lateral gutter adhesions, patellar entrapment from infrapatellar contracture syndrome, quadriceps contracture, reflex sympathetic dystrophy, and scarring postinfection.

Perform a thorough history and physical in order to determine whether there is an underlying cause to the arthrofibrosis. Radiographs help determine whether the tunnels are properly positioned or whether patella infera exists. Always rule out infection and CRPS. Aspiration of the knee as well as lab tests such as a white cell count, C-reactive protein (CRP), and sedimentation rate are helpful, though the erythrocyte sedimentation rate (ESR) and CRP may routinely be elevated for the first week after ACL reconstruction. An MRI helps determine whether a cyclops lesion is blocking full extension (Figure 27-1).

When discussing timing of surgery for motion problems, you must understand normal motion milestones and goals after ACL reconstruction. These milestones are not absolute, however, and a consistent progression of motion gains is more important than the actual motion limits. Alternatively, a distinct cessation of motion gains is worrisome and may dictate earlier surgical intervention. Avoid operating on knees with excessive warmth and inflammation, as further tissue scarring can result. A period of rest and avoidance of forceful motion combined with anti-inflammatory medication (NSAIDs [nonsteroidal anti-inflammatory drugs] and/or methylprednisolone dose pack) are indicated. An aggressive approach in patients with CRPS is to be avoided, as surgery may exacerbate the process. Treat the CRPS first.

Aggressive rehabilitation after ACL reconstruction emphasizes attainment of full hyperextension as soon as possible. Early active extension, full weight bearing in an extended braced knee, and active straight-leg raises help promote full extension. If your patient cannot do an active straight-leg raise at the initial postoperative visit due to a hemarthrosis, aspirate the knee. Attainment of full extension and 90 degree

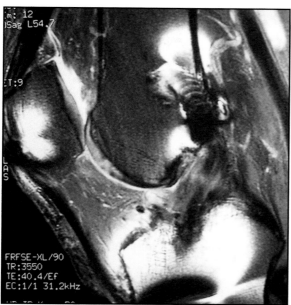

Figure 27-1. Sagittal T2-weighted image of a patient 3 years postoperative from a bone-patellar tendon-bone autograft ACL reconstruction. He had excellent stability but complained of pain and a feeling of hyperextension of the knee when he actively straightened his knee fully. Forced hyperextension caused retropatellar pain. He lacked just a few degrees of hyperextension. The MRI revealed scar tissue anterior to his ACL graft.

flexion by 2 weeks is the goal. If full extension is still lacking, prone heel hangs with or without weights as well as an extension board can be used. If at 1 week postoperative your patient attains those goals, he or she can return for a 6-week follow-up. If not, he or she should be seen 2 weeks later for a recheck with a goal of attaining full extension and 110 degree flexion. At 6 weeks postoperative full hyperextension and 125 degree of flexion should be present. If diminished patellofemoral mobility and poor flexion persists, consider using a methylprednisolone dose pack and continue with aggressive therapy including patellofemoral mobilization techniques. If 2 weeks later (8 weeks postoperative) there is less than full extension and 90 degrees of flexion, consider operative intervention. If motion is better than 0 to 90 degrees, continue with therapy and reassess in 4 weeks. At the 12-week postoperative period motion should be close to symmetric with the uninvolved knee, with a minimum goal of full extension and 130 degrees flexion. Consider arthroscopic lysis of adhesions at 12 weeks postoperative if less than 115 degrees of flexion is present.

Mild degrees of hyperextension loss are usually secondary to cyclops lesions.[4] Simple arthroscopic debridement is extremely efficacious in treating this problem (Figure 27-2). Extension loss greater than 10 degrees is likely due to an anteriorly positioned tibial tunnel.[5] Treat small losses of extension with debridement and notchplasty/roofplasty, but greater degrees of loss warrant an ACL revision. Conversely, an anteriorly positioned femoral tunnel causes loss of flexion or eventual graft elongation.

Whereas the arthroscopic treatment of extension loss is usually straightforward, arthroscopic treatment for flexion loss is more complex. Debride the scar tissue in the medial and lateral gutters and suprapatellar pouch first. Next, focus on debriding the scar tissue in the fat pad region so the normal space between the patellar tendon and anterior tibia is reestablished. More severe losses of flexion with patella infera require lateral and medial retinacular releases. Severe loss of extension may require open posterior capsular releases through meniscal repair approaches both medially and laterally. In general,

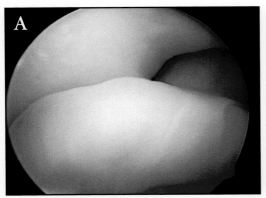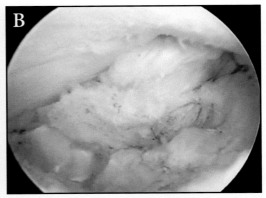

Figure 27-2. (A) Arthroscopic view of the intracondylar notch with the knee in near full extension. Nodular scar tissue is present and impinging. (B) View of the knee in full extension after successful debridement. At just 2 weeks postoperative, the patient had full hyperextension, no further feeling of hyperextension in active extension, and no pain with forced hyperextension.

the final motion gains are never better than what is obtained in the operating room. Fortunately, significant improvements in motion and subjective complaints are seen following arthroscopic debridement for arthrofibrosis.[6,7]

There are no hard-and-fast rules for determining the timing of surgery for motion loss after ACL reconstruction. In patients who are not reaching normal motion milestones after surgery, aggressive therapy and close biweekly evaluations are required. A plateau in motion gains warrants further arthroscopic intervention as long as the underlying cause of the motion loss does not preclude surgery.

References

1. Millet PJ, Wickiewicz TL, Warren RF. Motion loss after ligament injuries to the knee. Part I: causes. *Am J Sports Med.* 2001;29:664-675.
2. Millet PJ, Wickiewicz TL, Warren RF. Motion loss after ligament injuries to the knee. Part II: Prevention and treatment. *Am J Sports Med.* 2001;29:822-828.
3. Shelbourne KD, Patel DV, Martini DJ. Classification and management of arthrofibrosis of the knee after anterior cruciate ligament reconstruction. *Am J Sports Med.* 1996;24:857-862.
4. Jackson DW, Schaefer RK. Cyclops syndrome: loss of extension following intra-articular anterior cruciate ligament reconstruction. *Arthroscopy.* 1990;6:171-178.
5. Romano VM, Graf BK, Keene JS, et al. Anterior cruciate ligament reconstruction. The effect of tibial tunnel placement of range of motion. *Am J Sports Med.* 1993;21:415-418.
6. Klein W, Shah N, Gassen A. Arthroscopic management of postoperative arthrofibrosis of the knee joint: indication, technique, and results. *Arthroscopy.* 1994;10:591-597.
7. Noyes FR, Mangine RE, Barber SD. The early treatment of motion complications after reconstruction of the anterior cruciate ligament. *Clin Orthop Rel Res.* 277: 217-228, 1992.

WHAT CRITERIA DO YOU USE TO RETURN AN ATHLETE TO SPORT?

John-Paul H. Rue, MD, LCDR, MC, USN, and Brian J. Cole, MD, MBA

Determination of when an athlete may return to sport can be difficult, and there are many issues involved. There are 2 main issues that must be addressed prior to returning an athlete to sport. The first is biologic and relates to whether the graft fixation is stable and the graft itself has been reincorporated. This is typically accomplished at 5 to 6 months.[1] Bone-to-bone healing of autografts usually occurs by 6 to 10 weeks, but longer bone-to-bone healing rates of greater than 6 months have been reported due to slower incorporation in allografts.[1,2] There is no evidence that this delay in bone-to-bone healing has any detrimental effect on the strength of the allograft reconstruction. Both autografts and allografts undergo a process of ligamentization, and both initially decrease in strength and then subsequently undergo gradual increases in strength. This entire revascularization process typically occurs over a 5-month period. By 6 months, both grafts resemble normally oriented connective tissue, and histological studies have shown no difference in allograft and autograft bone-patellar tendon-bone grafts at 1 year.[3]

The second issue is the athlete's range of motion, strength, and coordination. This is very subjective and is also influenced by the level at which an athlete wishes to return to play. In general, in order for an athlete to return to sport, they must have regained full and unrestricted motion with strength equal to at least 85% of the contralateral side (Figure 28-1). Returning to sports participation prior to obtaining full and unrestricted range of motion places the affected extremity at a disadvantage mechanically and may increase the risk for further injury. We allow our patients to return to sports at 5 to 6 months postoperatively, provided that they meet the criteria shown in Table 28-1.

In a survey of members of the American Orthopaedic Society of Sports Medicine, most surgeons released their patients to competition at 6 to 7 months.[4] We believe that the graft is reincorporated and most patients have regained their motion and quadriceps strength by this time.

Figure 28-1. Complete quadriceps rehabilitation with symmetric tone and girth following bilateral anterior cruciate ligament (ACL) reconstruction.

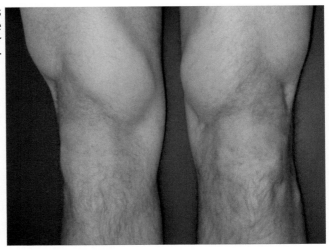

In order to return to sport, the athlete must progress through a dedicated rehabilitation phase of progressive sport-specific training. Sport-specific training simulates the functional requirements of the specific sport, simultaneously incorporating neuromuscular control and proprioceptive training. The athlete must be able to perform these complex drills prior to return to sport, as it is only through sport-specific training that he or she will develop the high level of reflexive neuromuscular control required to perform during competition.

Many athletes will bring up the question of bracing after anterior cruciate ligament (ACL) reconstruction. There is no definitive study showing any benefit to post-reconstruction ACL bracing. In a survey of members of the American Orthopaedic Society of Sports Medicine, 13% of 284 responders never braced their patients after ACL reconstruction and half braced their patients less frequently than 5 years prior,[5] possibly representing changes in rehabilitation protocols reflecting newer, more reliable fixation. Many surgeons do brace their patients for up to a year for sports; however, we do not feel that this is warranted except in rare cases or where the patients strongly request bracing for other subjective reasons.

Our rehabilitation protocol for return to sport progresses during the time period from 4 to 6 months. Patients progress with flexibility and strengthening and begin functional exercises such as running backwards, cutting, and pivoting. Plyometric exercise programs and sport-specific drills are initiated at this time as well. After 6 months, gradual return to sports participation is allowed and patients continue with a maintenance program for strength and endurance.[6]

In the end, the decision of when to return an athlete to his sport is a subjective one that is made after a thorough clinical evaluation, in conjunction with functional testing and subjective assessment of the athlete's overall progress. In my practice, I have found that presurgery discussions about an athlete's expectations of return to sport can be valuable tools in assisting me with this difficult question. Patients with realistic goals who are educated about the issues involved in returning them to sport can make more informed decisions about when they are ready and, probably more importantly, when they are not.

Table 28-1
Criteria to Return to Sport After Anterior Cruciate Ligament Reconstruction

Range of Motion	Strength	Duration of Time From Surgery	Rehabilitation
Full	At least 85% of contralateral side	Minimum 5 to 6 months	Must have completed entire rehab program, including sport-specific drills

Disclaimer

The views expressed in this article are those of the author and do not necessarily reflect the official policy or position of the Department of the Navy, Department of Defense, nor the United States Government.

References

1. Arnoczky S. Biology of ACL reconstructions. What happens to the graft? *Instr Course Lect.* 1996;45:229-233.
2. Markholf K, Burchfield D, Shapiro M, Cha C, Finerman G, Slauterbeck J. Biomechanical consequences of replacement of the anterior cruciate ligament with a patellar ligament allograft: II. Forces in the graft compated with forces in the intact ligament. *J Bone Joint Surg Am.* 1996;78:1728-1734.
3. Arnoczky S, Warren R, Ashlock M. Replacement of the anterior cruciate ligament using a patellar tendon allograft. An experimental study. *J Bone Joint Surg Am.* 1986;68:376-385.
4. Delay B, Smolinski R, Wind W, Bowman D. Current practices and opinions in ACL reconstruction: results of a survey of the American Orthopaedic Society for Sports Medicine. *Am J Knee Surg.* 2001;14:85-91.
5. Decoster L, Vailas J. Functional anterior cruciate ligament bracing: a survey of current brace prescription patterns. 284 responders. Half braced less frequently than 5 years prior. *Orthopedics.* 2003;26:701-706.
6. Cole B. ACL patellar tendon allograft/autograft reconstruction rehabilitation program. Available at: http://www.cartilagedoc.org. Accessed October 1, 2006.

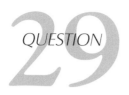

WHAT ARE YOUR EXPECTED RESULTS AFTER ACL RECONSTRUCTION?

Jerome J. DaSilva, MD, and Nihkil N. Verma, MD

The short answer is I expect the results to be similar between allografts and autografts. In my mind, the expectation that the results of allograft anterior cruciate ligament (ACL) reconstruction are similar to autograft ACL reconstruction must be a prerequisite for its inclusion in the informed consent discussion as a potential graft option for primary ACL reconstruction.

That being said, studies looking at allografts admittedly have shown high failure rates.[1-3] These studies suffer from poor study design, are not comparative in nature, and include sterilization techniques that often do not reflect the most current scientific knowledge. Roberts et al looked at freeze-dried, ethylene oxide–sterilized, bone-patellar tendon-bone allografts in 44 consecutive patients who underwent ACL reconstruction.[2] At 2-year follow-up, 8 cases of graft failure (18%) were confirmed arthroscopically. Pritchard et al looked at long-term follow-up of anterior cruciate ligament reconstruction using freeze-dried fascia lata allografts in 40 patients at an average of 134.5 months.[3] To the best of the authors' knowledge, no patients underwent a revision ACL reconstruction, although 19% fit the criterion for patient-reported failure (complaints of at least partial giving way episodes) and 7.7% had more than 5-mm side-to-side difference with KT-1000 arthrometer manual maximum testing. However, follow-up was not obtained on half of the subjects (49%); hence, lack of follow-up limits the ability to draw inferences from this study.

Contrary to many other studies showing higher graft failure rates for allografts, a study by Kustos et al showed similar graft failure rates for primary ACL reconstruction with fresh frozen, nonirradiated bone-tendon-bone (BTB) allograft and BTB autograft using the same surgical technique and postoperative rehabilitation.[4] In this retrospective clinical assessment, the groups were similar in age and activity level at baseline and at a mean follow-up of 38 months; both groups had similar (less than 4%) rates of revision ACL reconstruction; and there was no disease transmission attributed to the use of allografts.

In a quest to find the best available evidence on this topic, a literature search of manuscripts comparing bone-tendon-bone allografts to bone-tendon-bone autografts was performed. Using the keywords auto$.mp, allo$.mp, and Anterior Cruciate Ligament/ or acl.mp, Medline and EMBASE were searched (1950 to May 2007). Inclusion criteria were minimum 2-year follow-up, comparative study design, and the use of clinically relevant outcomes (Lysholm score, instrumented laxity, anterior knee pain, and/or graft failure). All studies were required to be level III or greater evidence and thus level IV studies were excluded. In the end, 8 studies, 4 level II and 4 level III, qualified based on the inclusion and exclusion criteria.[1,5-11] One comparative study by Gorschewsky et al was subsequently excluded due to the type of sterilization technique used.[1] The authors looked at the Tutoplast allograft, irradiated with 1.5 Mrad and subject to acetone solvent drying, versus the autologous patellar tendon in 201 patients (75% follow-up) at 2 years and 186 (69% follow-up) at 6 years following anterior cruciate ligament reconstruction. Failure rates were 20.6% at 2 years and 44.7% at 6 years for allograft patients, compared to 4.8% and 5.9%, respectively, for autograft patients. It is important to mention that the sterilization technique, acetone solvent drying, does not reflect current practices.

The following results are based on pooled data from the remaining 7 manuscripts comparing lower dose irradiation (less than 2.5 mRad) bone-tendon-bone allograft to autograft. Of the 6 studies that used instrumented measures of laxity, there were no significant differences between groups. Of the 5 studies that included the Lysholm, no differences were observed between allograft and autograft. Among the 5 studies that reported graft failure, the pooled bone-tendon-bone allografts failure was 5% to 6% compared with 1% to 2% for autografts. This slightly higher failure rate may be acceptable in many circumstances, especially if the patient understands this and still wishes to choose an allograft as his preferred graft option for other reasons. A high-quality randomized trial is necessary to determine whether there is a significant difference among allograft and autograft.

References

1. Gorschewsky O, Klakow A, Riechert K, Pitzl M, Becker R. Clinical comparison of the Tutoplast allograft and autologous patellar tendon (bone-patellar tendon-bone) for the reconstruction of the anterior cruciate ligament: 2- and 6-year results. *Am J Sports Med.* 2005;33:1202-1209.
2. Roberts TS, Drez D, Jr, McCarthy W, Paine R. Anterior cruciate ligament reconstruction using freeze-dried, ethylene oxide-sterilized, bone-patellar tendon-bone allografts. Two year results in thirty-six patients. *Am J Sports Med.* 1991;19:35-41.
3. Pritchard JC, Drez D, Jr., Moss M, Heck S. Long-term followup of anterior cruciate ligament reconstruction using freeze-dried fascia lata allografts. *Am J Sports Med.* 1995;23:593-596.
4. Kustos T, Balint L, Than P, Bardos T. Comparative study of autograft or allograft in primary anterior cruciate ligament reconstruction. *Int Orthop.* 2004;28:290-293.
5. Barrett G, Stokes D, White M. Anterior cruciate ligament reconstruction in patients older than 40 years: allograft versus autograft patellar tendon. *Am J Sports Med.* 2005;33:1505-1512.
6. Chang SK, Egami DK, Shaieb MD, Kan DM, Richardson AB. Anterior cruciate ligament reconstruction: allograft versus autograft. *Arthroscopy.* 2003;19:453-462.

7. Harner CD, Olson E, Irrgang JJ, Silverstein S, Fu FH, Silbey M. Allograft versus autograft anterior cruciate ligament reconstruction: 3- to 5-year outcome. *Clin Orthop.* 1996;Mar(324):134-144.
8. Kleipool AE, Zijl JA, Willems WJ. Arthroscopic anterior cruciate ligament reconstruction with bone-patellar tendon-bone allograft or autograft. A prospective study with an average follow up of 4 years. *Knee Surg Sports Traumatol Arthrosc.* 1998;6:224-230.
9. Peterson RK, Shelton WR, Bomboy AL. Allograft versus autograft patellar tendon anterior cruciate ligament reconstruction: a 5-year follow-up. *Arthroscopy.* 2001;17:9-13.
10. Saddemi SR, Frogameni AD, Fenton PJ, Hartman J, Hartman W. Comparison of perioperative morbidity of anterior cruciate ligament autografts versus allografts. *Arthroscopy.* 1993;9:519-524.
11. Victor J, Bellemans J, Witvrouw E, Govaers K, Fabry G. Graft selection in anterior cruciate ligament reconstruction—prospective analysis of patellar tendon autografts compared with allografts. *Int Orthop.* 1997;21:93-97.

IS THERE ANY SIGNIFICANT DIFFERENCE WHEN COMPARING THE RESULTS OF VARIOUS GRAFTS IN YOUR PRACTICE?

R. Edward Glenn, Jr., MD

The vast majority of anterior cruciate ligament (ACL) reconstructions I perform use ipsilateral patellar tendon or 4-strand hamstring autograft. I occasionally use patellar tendon allograft in revision cases or in patients over the age of 40 to minimize the morbidity of the surgical procedure. Other potential graft sources include contralateral patellar tendon, contralateral hamstring tendons, autograft quadriceps tendon, and various other allografts (Achilles tendon, tibialis anterior, quadriceps tendon, etc).

In my practice I have not found a significant difference in the final results of patients undergoing primary ACL reconstruction with either patellar tendon or 4-strand hamstring autograft. Range of motion, strength, stability, patient satisfaction, and return to sporting activity have been the same for both groups. These results parallel those found in the literature comparing patellar tendon and 4-strand hamstring autograft ACL reconstruction in prospective, randomized studies with a minimum 2-year follow-up.[1] It should be noted, however, that 2 studies comparing patellar tendon autograft to 4-strand hamstring autograft with greater than 3 years' follow-up demonstrated increased laxity in the hamstring reconstructed knees compared to the patellar tendon reconstructed knees.[2,3]

I discuss both graft options with all patients who require surgery for an ACL-deficient knee. I recommend patellar tendon autograft to all patients with sufficient patellar tendon width and whose occupation does not require excessive kneeling (ie, carpenter, carpet layer, roofer), as studies have shown an increased incidence of kneeling pain in patients who have undergone ACL reconstruction with patellar tendon autograft versus hamstring autograft.[1] In patients with a narrow patellar tendon width, I will recommend a hamstring autograft ACL reconstruction due to concerns of compromising the extensor mechanism with harvesting a 10-mm-wide patellar tendon graft. In patients whose occupation requires a lot of kneeling, I will also recommend a hamstring autograft for reasons cited previously. Finally, some patients will choose hamstring autograft over patellar tendon autograft for cosmetic reasons because the incision for hamstring autograft is significantly smaller than the incision for patellar tendon autograft.

Allograft ACL reconstruction makes up a very small portion of my practice. I try to use autograft tissue if at all possible. I will use allograft patellar tendon for primary ACL reconstruction in patients over the age of 40 who wish to minimize the morbidity of the surgical procedure. I have not seen a difference in the final results between autograft and allograft reconstruction, but the results in my practice may be biased because the patients receiving allograft tissue are older and typically less demanding than patients undergoing autograft reconstruction. A study comparing allograft and autograft patellar tendon ACL reconstructions in patients over the age of 40 demonstrated increased laxity and a higher failure rate in the allograft-reconstructed knees, but the differences did not reach statistical significance.[4]

References

1. Beynnon BD, Johnson RJ, Abate JA, Fleming BC, Nichols CE. Treatment of anterior cruciate ligament injuries, part I. *Am J Sports Med.* 2005;33:1579-1602.
2. Aglietti P, Zaccherotti G, Buzzi R, et al. A comparison between patellar tendon and doubled semitendinosus/gracilis tendon for anterior cruciate ligament reconstruction: a minimum five-year follow-up. *J Sports Traumatol.* 1997;19:57-68.
3. Feller JA, Webster KE. A randomized comparison of patellar tendon and hamstring tendon anterior cruciate ligament reconstruction. *Am J Sports Med.* 2003;31:564-573.
4. Barrett G, Stokes D, White M. Anterior cruciate ligament reconstruction in patients older than 40 years: allograft versus autograft patellar tendon. *Am J Sports Med.* 2005;33:1505-1512.

WHAT IS THE ROLE OF BRACING AFTER ACL RECONSTRUCTION, BOTH IN THE POSTOPERATIVE SETTING AND WITH RETURN TO COMPETITION?

James L. Carey, MD, and Kurt P. Spindler, MD

A systematic review of 12 randomized controlled trials (level I evidence) evaluated the use of bracing after anterior cruciate ligament (ACL) reconstruction.[1] The authors performed a quality appraisal of each original article and extracted data regarding type of brace, range of motion, instrumented laxity, activity level, knee scores, strength, functional testing, and complications.[1] The study concluded that there was no evidence to support the routine use of functional or rehabilitative bracing in a patient with a reconstructed ACL.[1] Specifically, no study demonstrated a clinically important finding of improved range of motion, decreased pain, improved graft stability, or decreased complications and reinjuries.[1]

However, postoperative bracing is recommended in the 3 following circumstances. First, if you have a partial (grade 2) or complete (grade 3) collateral ligament injury with ACL reconstruction, in order to prevent abnormal varus or valgus forces, a brace can be applied during the healing phase. Second, if the surgeon elects to use a femoral nerve block for postoperative pain control resulting in temporary quadriceps inhibition, then a brace or immobilizer is recommended until muscle function returns. Third, some surgeons, when performing concurrent meniscus repair, use a brace to control range of motion in the early postoperative time period.

Similarly, a functional ACL brace is not recommended routinely for return-to-play based on the following 2 primary reasons. First, no study has shown a benefit to using a brace to prevent ACL reinjury when returning to play. Second, a prospective multicenter cohort study determined that the contralateral normal knee is at a similar risk of ACL tear

(3.0%) as the ACL graft after primary ACL reconstruction (3.0%) at 2-year follow-up.[2] So perhaps the role of bracing after ACL reconstruction is the role of prophylactic bracing.

In fact, with respect to prophylactic knee bracing in sports, a prospective randomized study (level I evidence) examined the efficacy of a knee brace to reduce the frequency and severity of knee injuries in an intramural tackle football program.[3] The use of prophylactic knee bracing significantly reduced the frequency of medial collateral ligament (MCL) injuries that occurred.[3] A greater number of ACL injuries also occurred in the control group than in the brace group, but no statistical significance could be assessed because of a small sample size (despite 21,570 athlete exposures that were studied).[3]

Functional knee braces fail to completely reduce pathological translations and rotations due primarily to the soft tissue interposed between the braces and the target bones. Further, protective knee braces in general reduce speed and have a tendency to migrate, which affects their protective function.[4]

References

1. Wright RW, Fetzer GB. Bracing after ACL reconstruction. *Clin Orthop Relat Res.* 2007;455:162-168.
2. Wright RW, Dunn WR, Amendola A, et al. Risk of tearing the intact anterior cruciate ligament in the contralateral knee and rupturing the anterior cruciate ligament graft during the first 2 years after anterior cruciate ligament reconstruction: a prospective MOON cohort study. *Am J Sports Med.* 2007;35:1131-1134.
3. Sitler M, Ryan J, Hopkinson W, et al. The efficacy of a prophylactic knee brace to reduce knee injuries in football: a prospective, randomized study at West Point. *Am J Sports Med.* 1990;18:310-315.
4. Greene DL, Hamson KR, Bay RC, Bryce CD. Effects of protective knee bracing on speed and agility. *Am J Sports Med.* 2000;28:453-459.

SECTION IV

FAILED ACL RECONSTRUCTION QUESTIONS

WHAT ARE THE CAUSES OF ACL RECONSTRUCTION FAILURE?

Kyle R. Flik, MD

The etiology of anterior cruciate ligament (ACL) reconstruction failure can be categorized as being either traumatic or atraumatic (Figure 32-1). Traumatic failure can occur either early or late in the postoperative period. Early traumatic failure may occur if athletic participation is allowed prior to graft incorporation. Late traumatic failure is due to an injury that is of the same magnitude that would suffice to cause a primary ACL tear. Since the prevention of traumatic ACL failure is beyond the surgeon's direct control, of most concern are the atraumatic failures, which can be prevented or minimized. Unfortunately, atraumatic failures remain the most common category of ACL reconstruction failure, and surgeon error is implicated as the cause of these failures. Failures in this category can be minimized by the surgeon with careful preoperative diagnosis and attention to technical detail during surgery.

When I evaluate a patient with a failed ACL reconstruction, I look carefully first for an atraumatic etiology. These failures are the result of either preoperative diagnostic error or intraoperative technical error. Preoperative diagnostic error includes failure to recognize and treat concomitant injury to secondary and tertiary ACL restraints. While untreated patholaxity is a recognized cause of ACL reconstruction failure, the single most common cause of ACL reconstruction failure remains surgeon technical error, especially in tunnel placement.[1,2]

Determining the exact cause of failure begins with a thorough history and physical examination, followed by careful radiographic analysis. Many questions should be answered prior to physically evaluating the patient. How long ago was the index procedure and what technique and hardware was used? Is the patient complaining primarily of pain or instability? Does the patient describe a new traumatic injury in a previously stable knee, or was the patient experiencing giving way episodes all along since the index procedure? Did the patient have range of motion problems or difficulty regaining

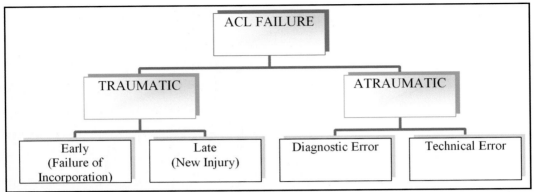

Figure 32-1. ACL failures defined by recurrent instability (not including complications such as infection or arthrofibrosis).

strength in the limb after the initial reconstruction? Review of previous operative records and images may also give clues as to the reason for failure.

During the physical examination, it is essential to evaluate the knee carefully to avoid missing concomitant injury to secondary or tertiary restraints to the ACL. Always examine the knee systematically and repeat the examination with the patient under anesthesia prior to surgery. Failure to recognize and address concomitant patholaxity may doom even a perfectly placed ACL graft.

Posterolateral instability, seen in 10% to 15% of chronically ACL-deficient knees, should be identified and treated if necessary.[3] Posterolateral instability is best identified by increased external rotation of the tibia with the knees bent at 30 degrees and is treated with concomitant posterolateral corner repair or reconstruction.

The medial collateral ligament and the posterior horn of the medial meniscus both provide secondary restraint to anterior translation.[4] Injury to either should be recognized and treated if appropriate in the ACL-injured knee. Medial meniscus insufficiency is diagnosed with magnetic resonance imaging (MRI) or from prior operative records and images. The meniscus may present as a treatable tear or chronic deficiency, which can be managed if needed with meniscus transplant surgery.

PCL insufficiency is best evaluated with a posterior drawer test at 90 degrees of knee flexion and a reverse pivot shift test and may be treated with posterior cruciate ligament (PCL) reconstruction.

Varus malalignment at the knee can also lead to chronic strain on and failure of the ACL graft. Mechanical alignment is best evaluated with standing weight-bearing hip-to-ankle radiographs and can be treated with high tibial osteotomy.

Radiographic analysis follows the physical examination in an attempt to identify the most common intra-operative cause of ACL failure, poor tunnel placement. Weight-bearing AP and lateral radiographs are best used to determine whether the tunnels are inadequately positioned. Proper tunnel placement is important in order to avoid excessive changes in graft length during knee range of motion or impingement on the intercondylar roof or the PCL, which leads to graft attrition.

Proper tibial tunnel placement is in the posteromedial aspect of the anatomic footprint so that it is parallel to Blumensaat's line on a full extension radiograph. An anterior tibial

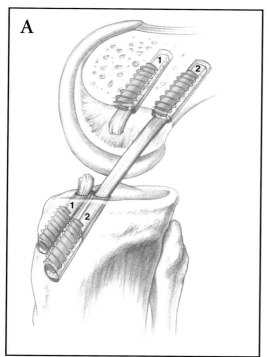
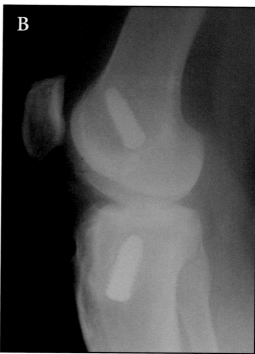

Figure 32-2. (A) Drawing of a graft placed too far anterior (1) revised with a graft (2) placed further posterior in a more anatomic location. (Reprinted with permission from Bach BR Jr, Mazzocca A, Fox JA. Revision anterior cruciate ligament surgery. In: Grana WA, ed. *Orthopaedic Knowledge Online*. Rosemont, IL: American Academy of Orthopaedic Surgeons; 2003.) (B) Lateral radiograph of a tunnel placed too anterior.

tunnel (Figure 32-2A) will lead to roof impingement and a flexion contracture. A tunnel placed too far posterior in the tibia will lead to a vertical graft that functions well to limit anteroposterior (AP) translation but functions poorly in terms of rotational stability. A medialized tibial tunnel will lead to graft abrasion from impingement on the PCL, and a lateral tunnel may impinge on the lateral notch. While proper femoral tunnel location is still debated, the most common error in tunnel placement is a femoral tunnel placed too anterior (Figures 32-2A and 32-2B), which leads to excessive tension on the graft in flexion and ultimately to failure. Femoral tunnel placement too vertical or too close to the center of rotation of the femur (Figure 32-3) will not reproduce normal knee kinematics, as rotational instability will remain. (Lachman test may be normal, but pivot shift test will be abnormal.)

With the single-incision endoscopic transtibial technique, surgeons may underestimate the effect that the tibial tunnel position has on femoral tunnel placement. Occasionally, I will place the femoral tunnel through an accessory inferomedial portal in order to locate it exactly where I want, rather than being restrained by the orientation of my tibial tunnel.

While proper tunnel placement can be difficult, nearly every step of ACL reconstruction surgery represents an opportunity for surgeon error. This begins with graft harvest. During this important step, the graft can be damaged, leading to weakness and failure. With patellar tendon grafts, an inadequate construct may be harvested. Attempts should be made to obtain a 10-mm-wide graft whenever possible, with bone plugs that are

Figure 32-3. Anteroposterior drawing of a right knee showing a vertically oriented femoral tunnel (1) revised to a more anatomic orientation (2). (Reprinted with permission from Bach BR Jr., Mazzocca A, Fox JA. Revision anterior cruciate ligament surgery. In: Grana WA, ed. *Orthopaedic Knowledge Online.* Rosemont, IL: American Academy of Orthopaedic Surgeons; 2003.)

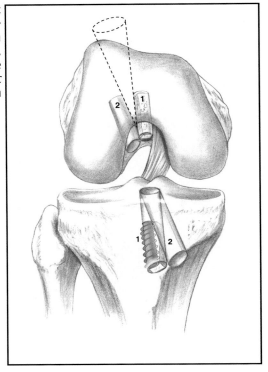

approximately 25 mm in length. Preoperative evaluation of the patient's patellar tendon width is necessary, so that if a narrow tendon (<25 mm) is present, hamstring autograft can be considered.

Poor fixation of the graft can also lead to failure. Interference screws, while stronger than staples or suture fixation around a post, do not provide adequate fixation if placed divergently.[6] For the femoral screw, I routinely use an accessory stab incision inferomedially to help orient the interference screw more parallel with the bone plug. Holding the hip in a flexed position while doing this will help as well. Finally, disruption of the graft may occur during placement of the interference screw, and care should be taken to protect the graft while advancing the screw.

References

1. Bach BR Jr. Revision anterior cruciate ligament surgery. *Arthroscopy.* 2003;19(suppl 1):14-29.
2. Johnson DL, Fu FH. Anterior cruciate ligament reconstruction: why do failures occur? *Instr Course Lect.* 1995; 44:391-406.
3. Gersoff WK, Clancy WG Jr. Diagnosis of acute and chronic anterior cruciate ligament tears. *Clin Sports Med.* 1988;7:727-738.
4. Harner CD, Giffin JR, Dunterman RC, Annunziata CC, Friedman MJ. Evaluation and treatment of recurrent instability after anterior cruciate ligament reconstruction. *Inst Course Lect.* 2001;50:463-474.
5. Bach BR Jr, Mazzocca A, Fox JA. Revision anterior cruciate ligament surgery. In: Grana WA, ed. *Orthopaedic Knowledge Online.* Rosemont, IL: American Academy of Orthopaedic Surgeons; 2003.
6. Kurosaka M, Yoshiya S, Andrish JT. A biomechanical comparison of different surgical techniques of graft fixation in anterior cruciate ligament reconstruction. *Am J Sports Med.* 1987;15:225-229.

WHAT ARE THE INDICATIONS FOR REVISION ACL SURGERY?

Shane J. Nho, MD, MS; Michael Pensak, BS; and John D. MacGillivray, MD

Current estimates show that approximately 100 000 new anterior cruciate ligament (ACL) reconstructions are performed annually in the United States, making it one of the top 10 most frequently performed procedures among orthopedic surgeons. Despite success rates reported in excess of 85%, ACL reconstructions do fail and a significant number of patients are left with unsatisfactory outcomes. A failed ACL surgery often culminates in a combination of the following morbidities: recurrent patholaxity, loss of motion/arthrofibrosis, painful arthritis, and extensor mechanism dysfunction. Typically, failures fall into one of the following 4 categories: technical errors, biological factors, trauma, and laxity of secondary restraints. Technical errors are responsible for roughly 70% of all failures.[1] Furthermore, over 75% of technical errors result from nonanatomical tunnel placement, specifically the femoral tunnel.[2,3]

The preoperative assessment of a patient who is a potential candidate for ACL revision is of utmost importance for several reasons. The physician must first determine whether or not the previous surgery has indeed failed because many of the persistent symptoms of a technically sound reconstruction can overlap and mimic the results of a failed graft. Next, it is essential that the physician differentiate the patient's primary complaint as either pain or instability. While both complaints may present with some degree of laxity on physical exam, the patient complaining of instability is more likely to benefit from an ACL revision than the patient complaining of primarily of pain. Pain can be caused by factors unrelated to laxity such as articular cartilage lesions or meniscus tears and therefore will not improve with a revision ACL reconstruction. Instability with activities of daily living or athletics and the presence of pathological laxity are the most important indications for a revision procedure. To sufficiently diagnose a failed ACL reconstruction, the following physical exam findings should be present: positive Lachman test with a soft endpoint, positive pivot-shift test, positive anterior draw sign, and maximum manual side-to-side difference greater than 5 mm as measured with the KT-1000 arthrometer. The medial and lateral secondary restraints must also be carefully assessed, and failure to identify laxity in collateral ligament structures can often mean the difference between a failure and success of a revision ACL reconstruction.

Radiographs are helpful in analyzing lower limb alignment, degenerative joint changes, bone quality, placement of hardware, tunnel placement, and tunnel enlargement. As such, a complete knee series including standing anteroposterior (AP), 45 degrees postero-anterior (PA) flexion weight bearing and lateral with knee in maximum hyperextension, notch, and Merchant views. Tunnel enlargement is best assessed with computed tomography (CT) images. Magnetic resonance imaging (MRI) should only be used to assess meniscal and articular surface status because the clinical exam and x-rays are sufficient to determine the status of the primary ACL graft.

The last portion of the clinical evaluation requires a straightforward explanation of the goals of the procedure and counseling the patient about realistic expectations. The physician should stress to the patient that revision ACL surgery is considered a salvage procedure to stabilize the knee, prevent further damage to the menisci and articular cartilage, and maximize the functional level of the patient. Patients should also be made aware of the fact that while revision has yielded good results with respect to improvement in instability, the results are not equivalent to those of primary ACL surgery. Candid communication will better prevent against false expectations for the revision surgery that may lead to a subjective feeling of failure in spite of a technically sound revision.

References

1. Bach B R Jr. Revision ACL reconstruction: indications and technique. In: Miller MD, Cole BJ, ed. *Textbook of Arthroscopy*. Philadelphia, PA: Elsevier; 2004:675-686.
2. Allen CR, Giffin JR, Harner CD. Revision anterior cruciate ligament reconstruction. *Orthop Clin North Am.* 2003;34(1):79-98.
3. Getelman MH, Friedman MJ. Revision anterior cruciate ligament reconstruction surgery. *J Am Acad Orthop Surg.* 1999;7(3):189-198.

HOW DO YOU MANAGE THE
EXPANDED FEMORAL OR TIBIAL TUNNEL
IN A FAILED ACL PATIENT?

Luke S. Oh, MD, and Thomas L. Wickiewicz, MD

Femoral or tibial tunnel osteolysis is a known phenomenon, particularly when soft-tissue anterior cruciate ligament (ACL) grafts are used. In revision ACL surgery, managing bone tunnels requires answering the following questions: (1) Is it possible to use the existing bone tunnels? (2) If not, is it possible to create new tunnels around the existing tunnels without overlap? (3) Does the previous fixation hardware need to be removed? (4) Do the tunnels need to be bone grafted? In cases of expanded bone tunnels, the answer to the first question is usually "no," and the majority of these cases will require a 2-stage procedure consisting of bone grafting and delayed revision ACL reconstruction.

Preoperative planning is essential for any revision surgical procedure, and revision ACL cases with expanded bone tunnels are no exception. If a reason for failure of the reconstructed ACL is not clearly evident, then a careful history and physical examination need to be conducted to evaluate for a possible complex laxity that was missed. If infection was suspected, appropriate serologic tests, imaging studies, and cultures need to be evaluated. Plain radiographs should be assessed for tunnel placement, tunnel widening, diameter and position of the fixation device, and bone quality. Magnetic resonance imaging (MRI) may provide additional information and is helpful to assess the amount and extent of tunnel osteolysis. Moreover, it may also identify pathology in the collateral ligaments, menisci, and articular cartilage. It is also important to obtain the operative report in order to identify the size, make, and model of the previous fixation hardware so that the appropriate hardware removal tray is available during the revision surgery.[1]

Despite diligent preoperative planning, the final decision to perform the revision ACL reconstruction in 1 stage or 2 stages will be dictated by the findings at the time of diagnostic arthroscopy, and the patient should be so informed. Depending on the location of the preexisting tunnels, it may be possible to create new tunnels away from the previous tunnels. For example, a preexisting tibial tunnel misplaced too anteriorly or posteriorly,

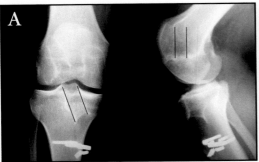
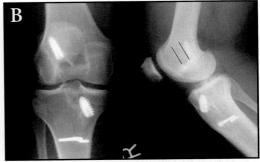

Figure 34-1. (A) An example of a tibial tunnel that was misplaced posteriorly with subsequent tunnel expansion and an anterior femoral tunnel. (B) Since it was possible to create new tunnels without overlapping the preexisting tunnels, a single-stage reconstruction with bone grafting was performed. (Radiographs courtesy of Bernard R. Bach, Jr., MD.)

Figure 34-2. (A) Since the position of the anticipated revision tunnels will overlap the preexisting expanded tunnels, the decision was made to proceed with a 2-stage procedure consisting of bone grafting and delayed anterior cruciate ligament (ACL) revision. (B) Radiographs after removal of femoral interference screw and bone grafting of both femoral and tibial tunnels with a composite graft consisting of tricalcium phosphate and autogenous osteoprogenitor cells from iliac crest bone marrow aspirate.

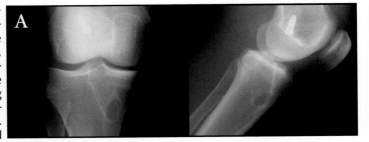
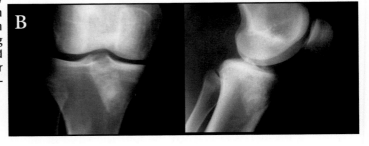

or a previous femoral tunnel misplaced too vertically or anteriorly may not overlap with an optimally placed new tunnel. Any fixation hardware that will not interfere with the creation of new tunnels should be left in place so as not to introduce a large bone defect. In such cases, a single-stage reconstruction may be performed (Figure 34-1). More commonly, however, the expanded tunnels will usually overlap the correctly placed revision tunnels. For these cases, a 2-stage procedure is recommended: the first stage consists of removal of any fixation hardware and bone grafting (Figure 34-2), and the second stage is a delayed revision ACL reconstruction after documentation of healing on imaging studies.[2]

During the first part of the 2-stage procedure, the goals include a thorough examination under anesthesia and diagnostic arthroscopy, exclusion of infection, evaluation and appropriate treatment of meniscal and chondral injuries, removal of the old graft, assessment of the notch, removal of any interfering fixation hardware, and bone grafting. It is our preference to use a synthetic bone graft substitute (eg, tricalcium phosphate or hydroxyapatite) in combination with iliac crest bone marrow aspirate. Although autogenous cancellous bone is considered to be the best bone grafting material, the procurement morbidity is a disadvantage. Synthetic bone grafts are good platforms for osteoconduction, but they lack any intrinsic properties of osteoinduction and osteogenesis. However, a composite graft that combines synthetic scaffold with autogenous osteoprogenitor cells from iliac crest bone marrow aspirate can deliver the advantages of autogenous bone grafts without the disadvantages. Other alternatives to autogenous cancellous bone from the iliac crest include demineralized bone matrices and freeze-dried allograft bone dowels.[3] Using an allograft may require a longer time to incorporate compared to an autograft.

The femoral tunnel should be grafted before the tibial tunnel. A graft protector may be placed in the knee through the anteromedial portal and used as a delivery tube to pass the bone graft to the entrance of the femoral tunnel. An alternative method is to use a chest tube, which allows visualization as the bone graft is pushed along the clear chest tube. Bone grafting of the tibial bone tunnel defect is easier since it can be done by direct visualization.

Depending on the size of the enlarged tunnels, bone quality of the patient, and type of bone graft used, the bone graft may take 6 to 12 weeks to incorporate. A computed tomography (CT) scan is recommended to evaluate and confirm incorporation of the bone graft prior to performing the delayed ACL reconstruction. The goal of the revision ACL reconstruction is the same as that of a primary reconstruction: select an appropriate graft and place it in an anatomic position in a good quality bone with adequate fixation.

References

1. Carson EW, Simonian PT, Wickiewicz TL, Warren RF. Revision anterior cruciate ligament reconstruction. *Instr Course Lect*. 1998;47:361-368.
2. Thomas NP, Kankate R, Wandless F, Pandit H. Revision anterior cruciate ligament reconstruction using a 2-stage technique with bone grafting of the tibial tunnel. *Am J Sports Med*. 2005;33(11):1701-1709.
3. Battaglia TC, Miller MD. Management of bony deficiency in revision anterior cruciate ligament reconstruction using allograft bone dowel: surgical technique. *Arthroscopy*. 2005;21(6):767.

WHAT GRAFTS DO YOU USE FOR REVISION ACL RECONSTRUCTION?

Scott A. Rodeo, MD

My choice is to generally use allograft tissue for revision anterior cruciate ligament (ACL) reconstruction. Allograft tissue has several specific advantages. Allograft provides availability of a large graft, which can be especially useful in the setting of bone tunnel enlargement. Bone deficiency may also be caused by removal of hardware or other fixation devices used for the primary ACL reconstruction. Allograft also eliminates donor site morbidity, which is more of a concern in revision ligament surgery where there is scarring from prior surgery. Patients undergoing revision surgery may have some degree of patellofemoral degeneration, making bone-patellar tendon-bone or quadriceps tendon-bone autograft less attractive. A further advantage of allograft is to decrease surgical time, which is relevant in revision ACL surgery since these knees often require additional meniscal or ligament surgery.

Previous studies by Noyes et al[1] reported relatively high failure rates using allograft for revision ACL reconstruction. One reason for these higher failure rates may have been from treatment of the allograft tissue with gamma irradiation. It is well established that gamma irradiation causes deterioration in biomechanical properties of tendon grafts in a dose-dependent fashion.[2] The availability of new proprietary sterilization methods for allograft tissue may allow a margin of safety while preserving normal biomechanical properties of the tissue.

I favor use of allograft tissue with attached bone (either bone-patellar tendon-bone or Achilles) if there is significant bone tunnel enlargement. Allograft tissue allows use of a large enough bone plug to address bone deficiency/tunnel enlargement. Careful preoperative imaging is critical to examine the position and size of the previous tunnels (Figures 35-1 and 35-2). A computed tomography (CT) scan may be helpful in this regard. If tunnel diameters are greater than 15 mm, I will consider a 2-stage procedure with bone grafting of the tunnels followed by revision ACL reconstruction 3 to 4 months later.

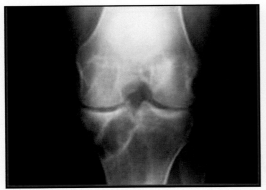

Figure 35-1. Anteroposterior (AP) and lateral radiograph showing significant tunnel widening of the tibial tunnel. This degree of enlargement would require a 2-stage procedure with primary bone grafting followed by second-stage revision reconstruction.

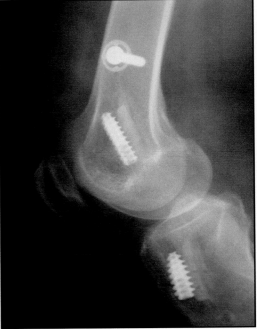

Figure 35-2. Lateral view showing anterior tunnel placement of femoral graft during index procedure.

The size and location of prior tunnels also helps to determine the best surgical approach for drilling new tunnels and inserting the revision graft, especially if a large allograft bone block is being used. For example, a 2-incision approach may be recommended to drill a new femoral tunnel if the primary reconstruction was done using a transtibial endoscopic technique. The graft should be inserted through the tunnel with the largest diameter, in order to accommodate a large allograft bone block. Thus, the graft would be brought in retrograde through the femoral tunnel (necessitating a 2-incision approach) if a large allograft bone block is being used to fill an enlarged femoral tunnel.

If there is no significant bone tunnel enlargement, a purely soft-tissue allograft such as tibialis anterior can be used. The advantage of this tissue is its robust size. A soft-tissue allograft should be fixed using a high stiffness, cortical-based device.

There are certain circumstances where autograft tissue can be used for revision ACL reconstruction. If a patient refuses use of allograft, I would recommend using either a bone-patellar tendon-bone graft or quadriceps tendon-bone graft. If a hamstring graft had been used for the primary reconstruction and preoperative imaging demonstrated that the tunnels were not excessively enlarged, a bone-patellar tendon-bone autograft would be recommended. I would not reharvest the patellar tendon if it had been used for the primary reconstruction. Autograft hamstring tendon would not generally be used due to the unpredictability in graft diameter, especially in the revision setting where a larger diameter graft is preferred. I recommend against using a graft harvested from the contralateral knee, although that would be a further option if ipsilateral autograft were not appropriate and the patient refused use of allograft tissue.

References

1. Noyes FR, Barber-Westin SD, Roberts CS. Use of allografts after failed treatment of rupture of the anterior cruciate ligament. *J Bone Joint Surg Am*. 1994;76(7):1019-1031.
2. Curran AR, Adams DJ, Gill JL, Steiner ME, Scheller AD. The biomechanical effects of low-dose irradiation on bone-patellar tendon-bone allografts. *Am J Sports Med*. 2004;32(5):1131-1135.

WHEN DO YOU USE THE CONTRALATERAL PATELLAR TENDON FOR REVISION ACL RECONSTRUCTION?

Nicholas T. Dutcheshen, MD, and Thomas J. Gill, MD

Revision anterior cruciate ligament (ACL) reconstruction can be challenging. Obstacles encountered during this surgery include tunnel malposition, tunnel widening, removal of retained hardware, bone loss, graft selection, and graft fixation. With reported failure rates of the primary surgery between 10% and 15%, we are performing an increased number of ACL revisions each year.[1]

Selecting the optimal graft for primary or revision ACL reconstruction is done during the preoperative planning. The decision is dependent upon patient age, previous graft used for the primary ACL reconstruction, surgeon preference/familiarity with the particular graft, and patient preference. Issues such as the presence of tunnel widening, the need to restore bone stock, the activity level of the patient, and history of preoperative anterior knee pain must also be considered.

Graft options for both primary and revision surgery include ipsilateral bone-patellar tendon-bone (BTB) autograft, contralateral BTB autograft, quadriceps tendon autograft, hamstring tendon autograft, and a host of allografts (eg, patellar tendon, Achilles tendon, tibialis anterior tendon). For ACL revisions, if a hamstring tendon autograft or an allograft was used for the primary procedure, we typically feel that an ipsilateral BTB autograft is the best option for graft selection in a patient younger than 40 years old. However, if the patient is older than 40, we prefer to use a BTB allograft for most procedures. In general, we do not like to use hamstring tendons for revisions, since there is typically some degree of tunnel widening present, and we have concerns about the ability of a soft-tissue graft to heal in a widened tunnel. Use of an allograft can allow for restoration of this bone stock. Moreover, if the patient had previously undergone the reconstruction using their ipsilateral patellar tendon, we do not feel that reharvesting the graft from the same location is a viable option and would thus use a patellar tendon allograft, regardless of age.

As a general rule, we do not ever use the contralateral patellar tendon for primary or revision ACL reconstructions. In our experience, the vast majority of complications following an appropriately performed ACL reconstruction are due to donor site morbidity. Thus, the logic behind harvesting the contralateral patellar tendon and jeopardizing the integrity and symptomatology of the "good knee" is not readily apparent. That having been said, there are theoretically some situations where its use may be indicated. For example, if the patient is philosophically opposed to allograft tissue and is undergoing a revision where the previous surgery utilized the ipsilateral patellar tendon, the contralateral patellar tendon may be an option. In addition, there are health care settings in which readily available, safe, cost-effective allograft tissue is not obtainable for revision surgery; therefore, harvesting the contralateral patellar tendon may be considered.

Advocates of using the contralateral patellar tendon cite several theoretical advantages to its use. First, it does lessen the surgical trauma to the knee that is undergoing the revision reconstruction. This may be potentially advantageous in regaining preoperative range of motion and quadriceps strength in a knee that has already undergone previous surgery. Second, this graft offers the advantage of secure bony fixation within the tunnels allowing more aggressive rehabilitation over other graft options. Finally, using autograft avoids any potential complications such as disease transmission that otherwise may potentially occur if one were to use an allograft.

In the literature, there are authors who advocate the use of a contralateral patellar tendon for ACL reconstruction.[2,3] These authors state that by dividing the trauma of surgery and the rehabilitation program between the 2 knees, the course of rehabilitation is easier, quicker, and more reliable. The authors promote using a contralateral graft in those athletes who require a safe and predictable return to sport, without compromising strength, range of motion, stability, and function.

We feel that there are many disadvantages of using the contralateral knee for graft selection. First, and most importantly, the surgeon violates a previously normal knee. This introduces a myriad of potential postoperative complications related to the donor site. These complications include infection at this site, anterior knee pain, quadriceps muscle weakness, loss of motion, patella fracture, patellofemoral crepitus, patellar tendonitis, and patellofemoral joint pain. Second, the operative time is longer, as the surgeon now has to prep and drape the contralateral leg, harvest the graft, and close the wound. Third, the patient will have scars on 2 knees instead of one. Fourth, it is not uncommon in certain patient populations to rupture the contralateral ACL following a return to sport. By harvesting the patellar tendon from the opposite knee, the surgeon no longer has the option of using that patellar tendon for the reconstruction. Finally, we feel that rehabilitation is more confusing for both the therapist and the patient as they now have different goals for each knee. Regardless of where the graft is harvested, it still takes the same amount of time to "heal" and mature in the knee—this is not a "pain-only" dependent factor. The immediate focus for the reconstructed knee is range of motion and the focus for the donor knee is strengthening.

Revision ACL reconstruction can be challenging. Like any ACL reconstruction, there are many decisions the surgeon must make regarding the surgical equipment, graft choice, and type of fixation used. There is no current consensus in the literature indicating that one graft choice is better than another. In most circumstances, we feel that a BTB autograft remains the gold standard for both primary and revision ACL reconstruction if the patient is less than 40 years old, although we are performing more primary hamstring reconstructions now that fixation techniques have improved. If the patient is older than 40 or has previously undergone an ipsilateral BTB autograft, we would most likely use an allograft patellar tendon. Based on the disadvantages previously stated, we do not recommend harvesting the contralateral patellar tendon for primary or revision ACL reconstruction unless options are severely limited.

References

1. Bach BR, Tradonsky S, Bojchuk J, et al. Arthroscopically assisted anterior cruciate ligament reconstruction using patellar tendon autograft. Five-to nine-year follow-up evaluation. *Am J Sports Med.* 1998;26:20-29.
2. Shelbourne KD, Urch SE. Primary anterior cruciate ligament reconstruction using the contralateral autogenous patellar tendon. *Am J Sports Med.* 2000;28:651-658.
3. Rubinstein RA, Shelbourne KD, VanMeter CD, et al. Isolated autogenous bone-patellar tendon-bone graft site morbidity. *Am J Sports Med.* 1994;22:324-327.

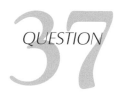

Is Your Rehabilitation Protocol Different in First Time Versus Revision ACL Patients?

Shane J. Nho, MD, MS; Michael Pensak, BS; and John D. MacGillivray, MD

Rehabilitation following revision anterior cruciate ligament (ACL) surgery can be different from protocols followed after primary reconstructions. In formulating a protocol the physician often has to take into account several surgical and patient variables that are unique to revision ACL surgeries so that a more patient-specific protocol can be developed. Moreover, the physician must discuss with the patient the expectations of revision ACL reconstruction, and the level of activity may vary on a case-by-case basis. Regardless, patients who elect to have a revision ACL procedure performed need to be highly motivated and adherent to their physical therapy so clinical and functional outcomes can be maximized.

The most common surgical variables that factor into a rehabilitation protocol following revision ACL surgery are strength of initial graft fixation, laxity of secondary restraints, associated ligamentous injuries, and the presence of more significant articular cartilage damage. The presence of any combination of the aforementioned issues may alter the intensity and course of rehabilitation.

Changes in the rehabilitation program following revision ACL surgery primarily consist of a slower progression to weight-bearing and functional exercises. Immediately following surgery, full passive extension to 0 degrees (avoiding hyperextension), actively assisted exercises using the opposite leg, heel drags, wall slides, quadriceps isometrics, straight-leg raises (quadriceps lag less than 10 degrees), ankle pumps and patellar mobilization are permitted. Restoration of full range of motion should occur by the sixth postoperative week. A hinged knee brace should be worn until the patient can display appropriate muscular control of the leg. In the absence of any associated ligamentous surgery at the time of the revision procedure, the maximum weight-bearing limit of the patient should be increased by no more than 25% of the patient's body weight per week. A gradual transition off crutches should begin no earlier than the fourth postoperative week and only if the patient is able to demonstrate normal or near-normal gait pattern with sound neuromuscular control of the leg. Stationary bike conditioning is encouraged as early as the fourth postoperative week and no later than the sixth week, at which time weight-bearing closed-chain exercises such as minisquats, lateral step-ups, toe raises, and the stair climber may begin. Jogging and running are delayed until 16 to 20 weeks after surgery while turning, twisting, and pivoting drills are delayed until the 24th postoperative week. Most patients are advised to avoid returning to pivoting sports until at least 9 months following their revision ACL procedure.[1]

Not all orthopedists are in agreement over which rehabilitation protocol to use in their revision patients. If the initial fixation of the graft is secure, several doctors are in favor of using their index ACL reconstruction protocol with their revision patients as opposed to more conservative and activity-delaying regimens. Some advocate a distinctly different rehabilitation scheme for their revision ACL patients. Postoperatively, patients are immediately permitted to bear full weight, unlock or remove their knee brace for range-of-motion exercises, discontinue the use of crutches by the first postoperative week if comfortable, begin bicycle riding by the second postoperative week, begin straight-ahead jogging by postoperative weeks 12 to 16, and gradually return to sports as early as 4 months postoperatively.[2]

References

1. Brown CH Jr, Carson EW. Revision anterior cruciate ligament surgery. *Clin Sports Med.* 1999;18(1):109-171.
2. Fox JA, Pierce M, Bojchuk J, Hayden J, Bush-Joseph CA, Bach BR Jr. Revision anterior cruciate ligament reconstruction with nonirradiated fresh-frozen patellar tendon allograft. *Arthroscopy.* 2004;20(8):787-794.

DOES HARDWARE HAVE TO ROUTINELY BE REMOVED AT THE TIME OF REVISION ACL SURGERY?

R. Edward Glenn, Jr., MD

Failed anterior cruciate ligament (ACL) reconstructions are attributable to technical errors at the time of the index procedure, repeat traumatic episodes, or failure of graft incorporation. Technical errors account for the majority of failures and include improper tunnel placement, improper graft tensioning, graft impingement due to insufficient notchplasty, failure of graft fixation, insufficient graft material, and failure to recognize associated knee pathology.

Improper tunnel placement is the most common technical error encountered in ACL reconstruction failures. It is critical to place the tibial tunnel at the appropriate angle in the coronal and sagittal planes during the index procedure to allow for appropriate femoral tunnel placement when the procedure is performed endoscopically. If the tibial tunnel is placed too anteriorly, excessive tension will be seen across the ligament in flexion and extension. The tibial tunnel placed too posteriorly will result in excessive laxity as the knee moves into flexion. A medially placed tibial tunnel will lead to impingement and subsequent friction between the reconstructed ACL and the native posterior cruciate ligament (PCL). A lateral tibial tunnel will result in abrasion of the ACL by the lateral aspect of the intercondylar notch, and this process is accelerated if an inadequate notchplasty is performed. On the femoral side, the tunnel can be placed too anteriorly, too vertically, or too posteriorly. If the femoral tunnel is too anterior, excessive tension is placed across the ligament as the knee is flexed. If the femoral tunnel is placed vertically, the reconstructed ligament will provide anterior to posterior translational stability but does not afford rotational control (Figure 38-1). This manifests as a normal or near-normal Lachman test but a positive pivot-shift test. If the femoral tunnel is too posterior, excessive stress is placed across the ligament as the knee is extended.

Prior to revision ACL reconstruction, a thorough preoperative evaluation of tunnel position is crucial. Previous operative notes and arthroscopic images are helpful, but

Figure 38-1. Arthroscopic image of a vertically placed graft. (Reprinted from Glenn RE Jr, Bach BR Jr. Technical aspects of revision ACL reconstruction. In: Freedman KB, ed. *Complications in Orthopaedics: Anterior Cruciate Ligament Surgery.* Rosemont, IL: American Academy of Orthopaedic Surgeons; 2005:61-73.)

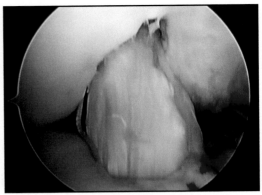

radiographic evaluation is essential and can often reveal the cause of graft failure. Standing anteroposterior (AP), 45 degrees flexion posteroanterior, lateral, and Merchant views are obtained. These radiographs can determine whether the previously created tunnels are in an anatomic or nonanatomic position. In addition, radiographs may also demonstrate tunnel widening, which may require bone grafting and a staged reconstruction.

The correct intra-articular entry and exit points of the tibial and femoral tunnels can be accomplished from various extra-articular tunnel paths. This is known as the divergent tunnel or "funnel" concept (Figure 38-2).[1] This concept is important to understand when deciding whether preexisting hardware needs to be removed. This concept may also help to determine whether the revision ACL reconstruction may be performed endoscopically or requires a 2-incision technique. For example, although the same femoral intra-articular entry point can be obtained using an endoscopic or 2-incision technique, the extra-articular femoral tunnel directions are quite different. Additionally, if the tibial entry point enters the joint in the appropriate intra-articular location, but the extra-articular tunnel is drilled too vertically, the corresponding femoral tunnel will also be placed vertically if an endoscopic reconstruction is performed. By orienting the tibial tunnel in a more medial to lateral orientation, the tunnel will still place the graft in the appropriate intra-articular location and will allow the femoral tunnel to be placed anatomically in the notch.

In general, 2-incision ACL reconstructions can be revised endoscopically, and the majority of endoscopic ACL reconstructions can be revised endoscopically. A 2-incision technique may be needed for a failed endoscopic ACL reconstruction secondary to posterior cortical wall blowout or overlapped tunnels that may affect graft fixation. The 2-incision technique will provide "tunnel divergence" for an intact tube of bone on the femoral side for adequate graft fixation.

If the prior tibial tunnel can be bypassed, hardware is left in place. If the hardware blocks the path of the new tibial tunnel, it must be removed. Fluoroscopy may be required to identify the previous hardware. If the tunnels overlap and do not have a sufficient bony bridge between the new and old tibial tunnels, the old screw may be temporarily removed and then replaced at the time of graft fixation to the tibia, essentially "stacking" the old and new interference screws. Alternatively, the old tibial tunnel may be bone grafted and a single interference screw may be used. If there is still a concern of adequate tibial fixation, a screw-and-post construct or use of a Hewson ligament button (Richards, Memphis, TN) may be employed.

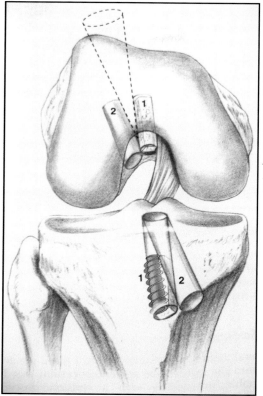

Figure 38-2. Diverging tunnel or funnel concept. Although both tibial tunnels have the same intra-articular entry point, the extra-articular paths are different. If tibial tunnel 1 is used to drill the femoral tunnel, the femoral tunnel will be placed too vertical. Tibial tunnel 2 is placed in a more appropriate orientation which allows for a more anatomic femoral tunnel placement. (Reprinted from Glenn RE Jr, Bach BR Jr. Technical aspects of revision ACL reconstruction. In: Freedman KB, ed. *Complications in Orthopaedics: Anterior Cruciate Ligament Surgery.* Rosemont, IL: American Academy of Orthopaedic Surgeons; 2005:61-73.)

If the femoral tunnel is in the appropriate location, it may be reused. If the femoral tunnel is in a nonanatomic position, the hardware may be bypassed and an entirely new femoral tunnel is created. If only the intra-articular entry point is in the appropriate location, the "diverging tunnel" concept is utilized. If the previous and current femoral tunnels are overlapping, bone graft is utilized to fill the defect left by the previous tunnel. Bone grafting of the femoral tunnel should be performed through a clear cannula and packed tightly into the tunnel to create a firm osseous tunnel. Other options include using larger bone plugs or "stacking" interference screws. In the case of a posterior wall-deficient femoral tunnel, a 2-incision technique should be considered.

References

1. Glenn RE Jr, Bach BR Jr. Technical aspects of revision ACL reconstruction. In: Freedman KB, ed. *Complications in Orthopaedics: Anterior Cruciate Ligament Surgery.* Rosemont, IL: American Academy of Orthopaedic Surgeons; 2005:61-73.

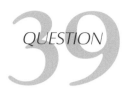

HOW DO YOU MANAGE THE PATIENT WHO HAS EARLY DEGENERATIVE JOINT DISEASE AND HAS COMPLAINTS OF PAIN AND INSTABILITY?

Annunziato Amendola, MD

First of all, the incidence and risk of degenerative joint disease of the anterior cruciate ligament (ACL)-deficient knee is significant, particularly with concomitant injury to the menisci and articular cartilage. In addition, a patient with predisposing factors such as preexisting varus alignment of the knee and who suffers ACL disruption may be at increased risk due to loss of some neuromuscular control of the knee.[1] This loss of control allows the knee to go into a little bit more varus and, therefore, overload the medial compartment with a higher risk of chronic medial compartment overload and degeneration. The ACL does provide neuromuscular feedback and mechanically does provide some varus control of the knee. Therefore, with chronic ACL instability, the development of further varus deformity will often result in further medial compartment overload. As a result, it is not uncommon to encounter patients who have early degenerative joint disease complaining of medial joint pain and overload as well as instability in the setting of ACL deficiency.

The typical wear pattern in these knees involves the medial compartment located more posteriorly on the tibial plateau. This occurs because of the chronic anterior subluxation of the tibia dynamically with respect to the femur. The wear pattern may be even further posterior in the setting of medial meniscal deficiency (Figure 39-1).[1] In addition, there is probably an age-related pattern in which the degeneration will be worse in the older patient population compared to the younger subacute and early post–ACL-injury group. As the arthritic changes in the medial compartment progress, the true instability of the knee usually becomes less of an issue due to the decreased motion, development of osteophytes, and contractures around the knee that occur with progressive arthritis. The instability symptoms from the ligamentous component become less prominent, although

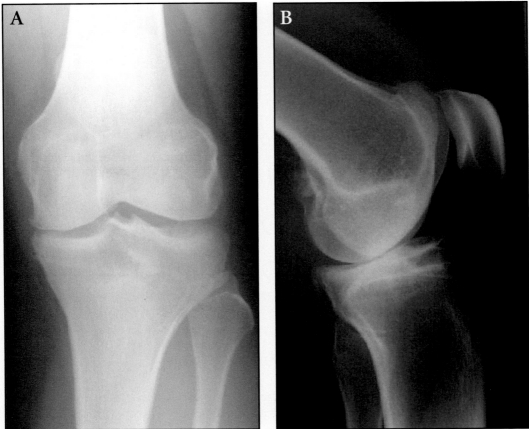

Figure 39-1. (A) AP x-ray showing medial comp narrowing, osteophytes, varus alignment 4 years post-ACL injury. (B) Lateral x-ray showing posterior subluxation of the femur on the tibia.

the patients may develop pseudo-instability symptoms from the arthritic change and catching from the irregularity of the degenerative joint surface. Therefore, the younger patient who has ACL instability with some degenerative joint disease likely has instability secondary to ligamentous laxity. The older patient who has more prominent arthritic change will likely be suffering more from the arthritic changes rather than the true ligamentous laxity.

In approaching these patients it is very important to clearly examine and delineate the problem that they are having with their knees. As mentioned above, it is important to outline what is giving them the symptoms—is it the actual giving-way and ligamentous instability or is it the painful problems from the degenerative joint disease, which may cause some symptoms of pseudo-instability? It is important to determine whether the degenerative change is only in the medial compartment versus the other compartments and whether the degenerative change is minimal or advanced. If the patients are having true ligamentous instability, then they will usually complain of this during more aggressive activities where the instability is evident, such as those involving some form of pivoting activity. Patients with isolated chronic ACL instability may have symptoms during

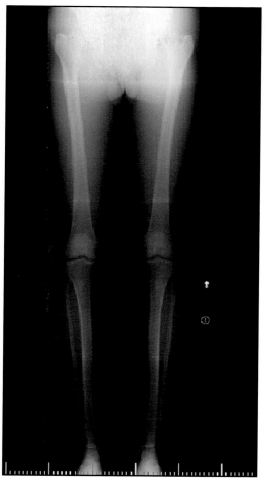

Figure 39-2. Double-leg standing demonstrating the mechanical axis in the med compartment in an ACL-deficient patient.

activities of daily living or straight ahead function, but this is unlikely. If they are having symptoms from those daily activities, it is important to rule out a degenerative meniscus or articular irregularity causing some sort of pain that leads to the instability episodes.

Putting this all together, a 25-year-old patient, for example, would be more likely to be unstable and have ligamentous laxity causing the episodes rather than the 45-year-old or older patient who has been chronically ACL deficient who is likely not as active, will not be stressing his knee, and probably will be suffering more from the degenerative changes of the knee rather than the ACL instability.

Imaging should include radiographic evaluation, including routine standing antero-posterior (AP) views of both knees, the flexed-knee standing view to outline the amount of articular cartilage wear, bilateral skyline, or Merchant views and bilateral long-leg views from the hips to the ankles to determine the mechanical axis deviation. It is important when taking the bilateral standing views from hips to ankles that the patient is standing comfortably and feet are pointed straight ahead and that the x-ray technician does not force him to put his knees together, which may reduce the true varus deformity (Figure 39-2).

If the patient then is diagnosed with a chronically ACL-deficient knee with some early medial compartment arthritis and varus malalignment with overload, the treatment would be to optimize a nonoperative regimen including muscular rehabilitation, reducing the pain and inflammation from the degenerative joint disease, or consider bracing with an unloader-type brace to unload the medial compartment as well as controlling the instability symptoms from the ACL. After these nonoperative options have been employed and the patient continues to be symptomatic, one could consider arthroscopic evaluation of the knee with debridement of any loose articular cartilage or degenerative menisci along with exam under anesthesia to determine the need for further surgery.

Typically, the type of patient that one will be faced with is the chronic ACL-deficient patient who may have had a partial medial meniscectomy and has mechanical axis deviation into the medial compartment with some early medial compartment degenerative change. In this situation, I would consider doing a high tibial osteotomy to correct the mechanical overload and treat the early degenerative change. I would do an arthroscopy at the time of the high tibial osteotomy and address any loose articular cartilage or menisci. I would consider a concurrent ACL reconstruction in the younger patient who is much more aggressive and does suffer from true instability. In general, in the older patient who is suffering from mechanical overload and pain, most patients respond well to osteomy alone, although ACL reconstruction can be considered as a secondary procedure if instability persists.

References

Clatworthy M, Amendola A. The anterior cruciate ligament and arthritis. *Clin Sports Med.* 1999;18(1):173-198, vii.

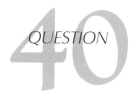

If You Have a Patient Who Is a Candidate for a High Tibial Osteotomy and ACL Reconstruction, Should You Perform a 1-Stage or 2-Stage Procedure?

Annunziato Amendola, MD

Before answering this question it is important again to emphasize that chronic anterior cruciate ligament (ACL) deficiency in active patients continues to lead to progressive deterioration of the articular cartilage of the tibio-femoral joint, most commonly the medial compartment. Patients who have had a previous medial meniscectomy or have preexisting varus are at higher risk of the progression of medial compartment arthritis. The outcomes following ACL reconstruction in ACL-deficient patients have demonstrated adequate control of anterior translation; however, in patients who present with chronic ACL deficiency with early arthritis, isolated ACL reconstruction alone probably does not prevent the progression of further arthritis, particularly if the patient remains active and continues in pivoting sports. High tibial osteotomy (HTO) in patients with early medial compartment arthrosis has been shown to be an effective method of reducing symptoms and possibly reducing the progression of osteoarthritis in these patients.[1] Patients who present with both ACL deficiency and malalignment with medial compartment overload have been shown to benefit from high tibial osteotomy and ACL reconstruction in both a 1-stage or 2-stage procedure.[1-5] Whether these procedures should be performed in these types of patients in a 1-stage or 2-stage fashion still remains controversial because of the technical difficulty of performing the 1-stage procedure as well as the additional possible risk of increased morbidity by performing both procedures at the same time.

Before deciding on performing a 1-stage or a 2-stage procedure, it is important to outline the symptoms of the patient. Generally speaking, the younger the patient, the more active the patient will be and the more likely that he will have some symptoms of true instability from the ACL deficiency despite the presence of some early joint degeneration. As the patient gets older and the severity of arthritis increases, the symptoms are probably going to be more due to the arthritis. Therefore, in general, the older patient with more advanced arthritis who is suffering more from arthritic symptoms would benefit the most from having the joint realigned and the degenerative compartment unloaded with a high tibial osteotomy. Latterman and Jakob used 40 years of age as the cutoff.[2] Many of these patients would do very well with the osteotomy alone and do not require any subsequent stabilization for the ACL deficiency. In addition, at the time of the osteotomy it is important to reduce the tibial slope because this will help in the anterior translation of the tibia and the chronic ACL instability.[1]

The younger patient who has some early degeneration with malalignment and ACL deficiency, and who has complaints of both pain and instability, would benefit from both procedures. In this type of patient, the question is whether you should utilize a 1-stage or 2-stage approach. In my opinion, it does not make any sense to do the ACL reconstruction alone. I think it is important to consider doing a high tibial osteotomy to unload the medial compartment as a definite component of the procedure. If performed as a staged procedure, the HTO should be performed first. Interestingly many of these patients will have elimination of symptoms following the performance of the osteotomy and realignment. However, in the younger patient my preference would be to do both procedures at the same time. The technical details of performing concomitant ACL reconstruction and HTO are outlined in another question. In my experience, using contemporary techniques, a single-stage procedure can be reliably completed with minimal morbidity.

Multiple authors have described a 1-stage approach with good outcomes. On the other hand, in one study by Noyes et al,[5] the author performed the HTO first[1,3,4] and subsequently performed an ACL reconstruction at 8 months following the procedures with similarly good results. Therefore, either a 1-stage or 2-stage procedure can be performed with good outcome, with the choice based primarily on surgeon preference. It is important to emphasize that the realignment procedure to unload the affected compartment should be performed as the minimum surgical treatment or as the initial procedure in a staged approach. The ACL reconstruction either at the same time or as a second-stage procedure should be secondary. Doing the ACL reconstruction alone will lead to inferior results and progression of the osteoarthritic change.

References

1. Bonin N, Ait Si Selmi T, Donell ST, Dejour H, Neyret P. Anterior cruciate reconstruction combined with valgus upper tibial osteotomy: 12 years follow-up. *Knee.* 2004;11:431-437.
2. Lattermann C, Jakob RP. High tibial osteotomy alone or combined with ligament reconstruction in anterior cruciate ligament-deficient knees. *Knee Surg Sports Traumatol Arthrosc.* 1996;4(1):32-38.
3. Dejour H, Neyret P, Boileau P, Donell ST. Anterior cruciate reconstruction combined with valgus tibial osteotomy. *Clin Orthop Relat Res.* 1994;299:220-228.
4. Williams RJ III, Kelly BT, Wickiewicz TL, Altchek DW, Warren RF. The short-term outcome of surgical treatment for painful varus arthritis in association with chronic ACL deficiency. *J Knee Surg.* 2003;16(1):9-16.
5. Noyes FR, Barber-Westin SD, Hewett TE. High tibial osteotomy and ligament reconstruction for varus angulated anterior cruciate ligament-deficient knees. *Am J Sports Med.* 2000;28:282-296.

WHAT TECHNICAL PEARLS DO YOU HAVE WHEN PERFORMING A SINGLE-STAGE ACL RECONSTRUCTION AND HIGH TIBIAL OSTEOTOMY?

Annunziato Amendola, MD

The preoperative planning and assessment of the patient is very important. As discussed in questions 39 and 40, it is important to understand the indications for the surgery and educate the patient about the condition of the knee joint, the malalignment, and overload in addition to the concurrent instability. Patients need to be clear on the procedure that is being performed and that the rehabilitation and weight bearing will depend on the healing of the high tibial osteotomy. Because of the concurrent anterior cruciate ligament (ACL) reconstruction, it will be important to begin early range of motion to prevent stiffness in the knee joint.

As part of the preoperative plan, it is important to assess preoperative alignment and plan the surgery in terms of the amount of correction required, the type of osteotomy that is going to be performed, and the type of ACL surgery that will be conducted for the reconstruction. Opening or closing wedge valgus tibial osteotomy techniques may be used. I prefer an opening wedge technique because it is simpler, allows for medial access for the ACL procedure of hamstring harvest, and allows performing the correction in 2 planes. It is my preference to use allograft soft tissue, preferably a tibialis graft, and do a single-tunnel ACL reconstruction (Figure 41-1). Hamstring autograft may also be used easily since the incision for the tibial osteotomy will be right there where the hamstring origin is on the tibia. The semi-tendinosis and gracilis can be harvested at the same time and used doubled, creating 4 strands and a very good graft for the reconstruction. For this procedure the patient will be admitted at least overnight for pain control and to begin early range of motion. The postoperative care will be in a hinged knee brace allowing

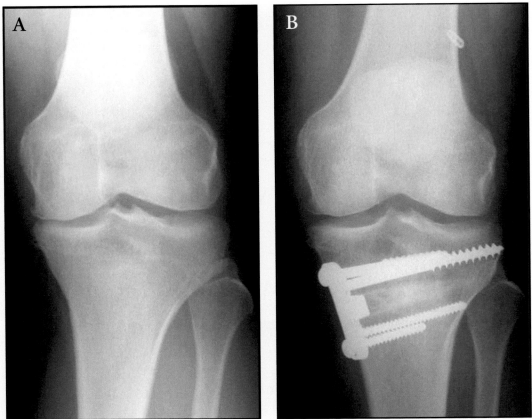

Figure 41-1. (A) Pre-ACL reconstruction and high tibial osteotomy (HTO) and (B) post-ACL reconstruction and HTO at the same stage.

90° range of motion, touch or non-weight-bearing with crutches for at least 6 weeks. Evaluation of osteotomy healing on radiographs at 6 weeks will determine progression of weight-bearing status. If everything looks good at 6 weeks and there is evidence of early x-ray healing, then begin 50% weight bearing for 2 to 3 weeks and then increase to full weight bearing after that. Strengthening exercises can begin around 6 weeks. Range of motion exercises, passive and active assisted, without resistance, begin at time zero up to 90° for 6 weeks and then full range of motion after the 6-week period.

The technical performance of the surgery is as follows: first the arthroscopy is performed, including any meniscal or articular cartilage surface work and notch preparation. In general, I do not perform articular cartilage resurfacing procedures, such as autologous cartilage implantation (ACI) or meniscal transplants, at the same time as this surgery. If these procedures are required, I will perform the realignment osteotomy first and do the soft-tissue procedures as a second stage once the patient has recovered from the osteotomy.

Once the knee joint is prepared arthroscopically, the incision is made and the osteotomy is performed. My preference is to perform the osteotomy first to prevent a possible stress riser through the ACL tunnel or to disrupt the ACL tibial tunnel with the osteotomy. My preference is to perform an opening wedge from the medial side; therefore, the

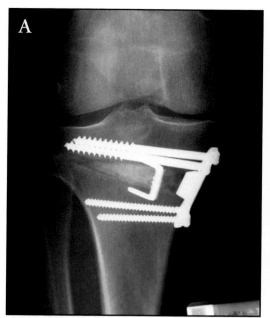 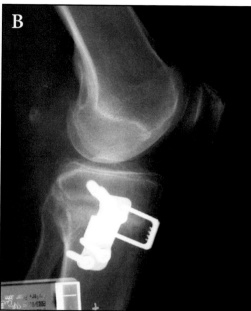

Figure 41-2. (A, B) Postop anteroposterior (AP) and lateral x-ray. Note that the plate is placed as posterior as possible, with the staple on the front to close the osteotomy anteriorly to decrease the anterior tibial slope.

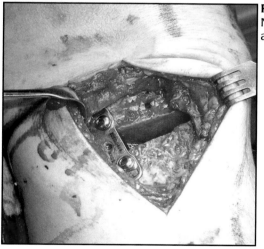

Figure 41-3. The plate is as posterior as possible. Note the closing of the wedge as it comes more anterior.

opening has to be directed from medial to lateral. At the time of fixation you should place a bump underneath the leg in order to hyperextend at the knee and close the osteotomy site anteriorly (Figure 41-2). This is very important to decrease the tibial slope to decrease anterior tibial translation in the ACL-deficient knee. The osteotomy is then fixed with the plate posteromedially and preferably some fixation anteriorly to create an anterior hinge either a staple, as shown in Figure 41-2, or a 2-hole plate (Figure 41-3). A wedged toothed plate is used to help decrease the risk of increasing the anterior opening of the osteotomy (Figure 41-4).

Figure 41-4. Angle wedge plates are used to help decrease tibial slope anteriorly.

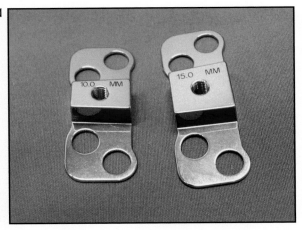

At this point, the ACL reconstruction is completed. The tibial tunnel is drilled, preferably exiting just above the osteotomy site anteromedially. A femoral tunnel is drilled in the usual technique. The ACL graft is passed through the tibia joint and out the femur. My preference is to use extracortical button fixation, either with a RetroButton or EndoButton. Fixation on the tibial side is with interference screw fixation above the osteotomy site and then secondary fixation can be placed below the osteotomy site if desired. Bone grafting of the osteotomy site is performed at this point.

In summary, the key to the performance of this procedure is the preoperative planning and education of the patient. Technically, the osteotomy is performed with the aim of reducing the tibial slope so that this will help the ACL reconstruction.[1] The ACL tibial tunnel is prepared after the osteotomy in order to prevent a stress riser during the osteotomy. Postoperatively, rehabilitation depends on the healing of the osteotomy site, but early range of motion must be started to prevent stiffness of the knee joint.

References

1. Agarwal A, Panarella L, Amendola A. Considerations for osteotomy in the ACL deficient knee; review article. *Sports Med Arthrosc Rev.* 2005;13(2):109-115.

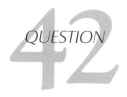

How Do You Manage the Postoperative Patellar Fracture Following ACL Reconstruction With Patellar Tendon Autograft?

Matthew Busam, MD, and Bernard R. Bach, Jr., MD

A postoperative patella fracture in the setting of a bone-patellar tendon-bone auto-graft anterior cruciate ligament (ACL) reconstruction can be a devastating complication. Prevention of patella fractures is key, but if one occurs, early recognition and prompt treatment provide the possibility of excellent results.

Patella fractures can be initiated intraoperatively during harvest of the autograft. The surgeon must avoid plunging with the saw, which could compromise cortical integrity. Forceful levering of the graft from its bed could propagate a fracture. Arthroscopic evaluation of the articular surface of the patella should always be undertaken after graft harvest in order to rule out a fracture as the result of harvest. Intraoperative fractures typically occur in the sagittal plane and require fixation perpendicular to the split (Figure 42-1). If the fracture is noted during the course of the procedure, immediate fixation may allow the patient to participate in the standardized aggressive rehab program.[1]

Postoperative fractures occur with 1 of 2 possible mechanisms. A direct blow results in an impaction injury, with the fracture being stellate or Y-shaped. A rapid eccentric quadriceps contraction, which may occur as the result of a fall, typically results in a transverse fracture pattern. These fractures occur relatively early in the postoperative time period, typically between 6 weeks and 6 months. Patella fractures are rare, with large series reporting only 3 in 1320 patients[2] and 8 in 2300.[3] Our experience is similar, with just one postoperative fracture in over 1700 bone-patellar tendon-bone (BTB) autograft ACL reconstructions performed by the 3 senior surgeons at our institution. Several factors contribute to the low number of fractures despite large numbers of BTB autografts. The

Figure 42-1. Intraoperative fracture in the sagittal plane with fixation perpendicular to the split.

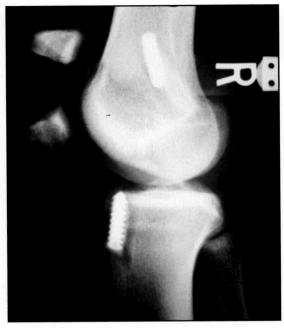

first is the inherent durability of the patella, even with a 25-mm cortical-cancellous plug harvested distally. Bone grafting the patellar defect also aids in restoring patellar stability as it incorporates. We use a cannulated bone chip collector during reaming of the tibial tunnel and make a concerted effort to collect reamings from the femoral tunnel as well. These are then grafted in the patellar defect. Furthermore, most ACL reconstructions are performed in patients who are younger, with excellent bone density. In addition, protecting the extensor mechanism in the early postoperative period is beneficial. While bracing is not likely needed to protect the graft,[4] a hinged brace, locked in extension for ambulation, protects the patella should a fall occur. The patient removes the brace for range-of-motion exercises and during physical therapy sessions. While many advocate a brace-free rehab protocol, our use of the brace is principally to protect the extensor mechanism in an attempt to avoid catastrophic failure. One must have a low threshold to obtain radiographs because patella fractures can present with documented fracture fixation stability and an intact extensor mechanism in this population.[5]

Patella fractures occurring outside of ACL reconstruction typically occur in middle-aged and osteopenic patients. Rigid fixation to allow early mobilization is the recommended treatment for most isolated patella fractures.[6] The same treatment goals are true for patella fractures in the postoperative period after ACL reconstruction. Nonoperative treatment and treatments requiring extended immobilization should be reserved for those patients unwilling or unable to undergo surgery or for a fracture pattern that cannot be rigidly fixed. Once a patella fracture occurs, the short-term rehabilitation goals for the patient need to be altered in order to preserve the likelihood of long-term success. Fracture healing without displacement becomes paramount. A variety of fixation methods exist. Tension-band fixation has been reported with successful results;[2] however, as reported in the trauma literature, 22% of patients treated with tension-band wiring and early motion had displacement of 2 or more mm, and just over 10% of patients will request hardware removal due to overlying irritation from the wire.[7] Other options include cannulated screw fixation, with or without a tension band augment or bicortical (superior to inferior) small or large fragment screw fixation. Biomechanical testing of a modified tension band vs 4.5-mm screws vs an anterior tension band placed through 4.0-mm cannulated screws showed that the cannulated screws plus tension band to be the strongest construct.[8] No matter which method is selected, the surgeon must achieve reduction of the articular surface with stability through range of motion. Once the fracture is reduced and stabilized, the knee must be taken through a range-of-motion to ensure that no displacement is noted prior to closure. Postoperatively, the patient is allowed protected progressive range of motion in a brace, but weight bearing is allowed only in full extension. In addition, the brace must be locked in extension during sleep. Beginning at the first postoperative visit, range of motion can begin from 0 to 60 degrees, with a goal of 0 to 90 degrees by 6 weeks. Aggressive, forceful flexion, even in supervised therapy, must be avoided until fracture consolidation is noted radiographically. The patient must be thoroughly counseled to ensure that the protocol is followed, because noncompliance is associated with failure of fixation.[7] Hardware should not be routinely removed,[9] but if symptomatic, it can be retrieved after the fracture is healed and ACL rehab is complete.

In general, postoperative patella fractures are extremely rare. The incidence can be further reduced with careful surgical technique and protection of the extensor mechanism postoperatively. If a fracture occurs, rigid fixation and an altered rehab protocol can allow excellent results.

References

1. Berg EE. Management of patella fractures associated with central one third bone-patella tendon-bone autograft ACL reconstructions. *Arthroscopy*. 1996;12(6):756-759.
2. Viola R, Vianello R. Three cases of patella fracture in 1,320 anterior cruciate ligament reconstructions with bone-patellar tendon-bone autograft. *Arthroscopy*. 1999;15(1):93-97.
3. Bear BJ, Cohen SB, Bowen MK, Siegel J, Moorman CT III, Warren RF. Fractures of the patella following anterior cruciate ligament reconstructions with the central one-third of the patella tendon. Paper presented at: Annual meeting of the American Academy of Orthopaedic Surgeons, Atlanta, GA, 1996.
4. McDevitt ER, Taylor DC, Miller MD, Gerber JP, Ziemke G, Hinkin D, Uhorchak JM, Arciero RA, St. Pierre P. Functional bracing after anterior cruciate ligament reconstruction: a prospective, randomized, multicenter study. *Am J Sports Med*. 2004;32:1887-1892.
5. Carreira DA, Fox JA, Freedman KB, Bach BR Jr. Displaced nonunion patellar fracture following use of a patellar tendon autograft for ACL reconstruction. *J Knee Surg*. 2005;18(2):131-134.
6. Mills WJ, Roberts CS, Miranda MA. Knee injuries. In: Baumgaertner M, Tornetta P, eds. *Orthopaedic Knowledge Update: Trauma 3*. Rosemont, IL: American Academy of Orthopaedic Surgeons; 2005.
7. Smith ST, Cramer KE, Karges DE, Watson JT, Moed BR. Early complications in the operative treatment of patella fractures. *J Orthop Trauma*. 1997;11:183-187.
8. Carpenter JE, Kasman RA, Patel N, Lee ML, Goldstein SA. Biomechanical evaluation of current patella fracture fixation techniques. *J Orthop Trauma*. 1997;11:351-356.
9. Busam ML, Esther RJ, Obremskey WT. Hardware removal: indications and expectations. *J Am Acad Ortho Surg*. 2006;14:113-120.

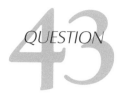

How Do You Evaluate Tunnel Position in the Revision Setting?

L. Pearce McCarty, III, MD, and Aimee S. Klapach, MD

Given that tunnel malposition accounts for an estimated 70% to 80% of anterior cruciate ligament (ACL) graft failures, evaluation of tunnel position in the setting of revision reconstruction is perhaps the most important element of preoperative planning.[1,2] Tunnel malposition can theoretically lead to graft failure through a variety of mechanisms, including impingement on the notch, posterior cruciate ligament (PCL), and lateral wall; development of abnormal tensile forces leading to graft elongation; and interference with normal knee motion via "capture." The issue of appropriate tunnel position has become particularly complex with the introduction and increasing utilization of double-bundle reconstruction techniques, and although a detailed discussion of ideal tunnel position in the context of ACL reconstruction lies beyond the scope of this text, we hope to provide at least a basic framework for approaching this difficult question in the revision setting.

Appropriate evaluation of tunnel position requires not only adequate radiographic delineation of tunnel location in the femur and tibia but also accurate correlation between tunnel position and etiology of failure. We therefore consider patient history and physical exam to be important adjuncts to radiographic and arthroscopic evaluation of tunnel position and in answering the following questions:

1. Is apparent tunnel malposition the primary cause of graft failure?

2. What is the nature of tunnel malposition (ie, is the femoral tunnel too anterior? Is the tibial tunnel too posterior?)?

3. Can the malpositioned tunnel be repositioned in a single setting and, if so, can it be bypassed entirely or does it constitute a "near miss" that needs to be grafted?

In regard to patient history, if the failure has an apparent traumatic etiology, did the patient experience recurrent instability prior to the recounted traumatic event? Did the patient have significant motion loss postoperatively? Did the patient have recurrent

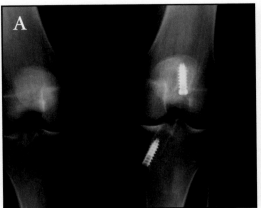
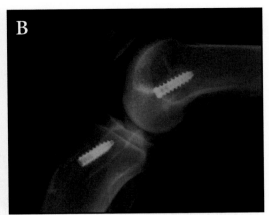

Figure 43-1. Anteroposterior (AP) and lateral radiographs of a patient with recurrent instability following anterior cruciate ligament reconstruction. Screw divergence, (A) midline (near 12 o'clock) and (B) slightly anterior position, is noted with respect to the femoral tunnel. Tunnel widening is noted on the tibial side.

discomfort or swelling postoperatively? Affirmative responses to any of these questions may suggest tunnel malposition as a causative element in failure of the index reconstruction.

We also find physical exam to be helpful in confirming apparent radiographic tunnel malposition as contributing to graft failure. For example, the finding of a pivot shift together with a grade I or II Lachman and a firm endpoint may suggest that a vertical-appearing femoral tunnel has controlled anterior-posterior translation but failed to correct rotatory instability and is therefore the principal etiology of failure.

Radiographic evaluation begins with a plain radiograph series consisting of a weight-bearing anteroposterior (AP), weight-bearing 45 degrees flexed posteroanterior (PA), and lateral. When a soft-tissue graft has been utilized for the index reconstruction, tunnel position is readily observable on plain radiographs (Figure 43-1). Use of grafts with bone blocks at one or both ends, however, may prevent accurate identification of bone tunnels. We are wary of accepting radiographic screw position as indicative of tunnel position, as—particularly on the femoral side—screw divergence may be present. In the coronal plane we look for the femoral tunnel to exit the lateral wall of the intercondylar notch at the 10:30 position on the left, and at the 1:30 position on the right.[3] On the tibial side we look for the tunnel to exit the tibial plateau along the lower one-third of the medial tibial spine (relatively central) and to make an angle of approximately 70 degrees with the joint line, particularly when endoscopic technique has been utilized and the femoral tunnel has been drilled through the tibial tunnel.[4,5] If a 2-incision technique has been used or the femoral tunnel has been drilled through an accessory portal, then the angle of the tibial tunnel in the coronal plane may be of less consequence.

In the sagittal plane we look for the femoral tunnel to lie near the posterior cortex of the femur. On the tibial side we look for a line parallel to the path of the tibial tunnel to lie just posterior to Blumensaat's line with the knee in full extension. At this time we also attempt to determine whether the malpositioned tunnel can be ignored at the time of

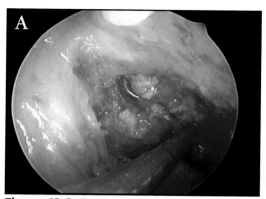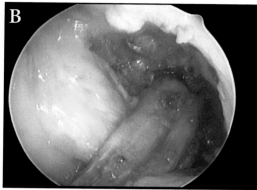

Figure 43-2. Intraoperative arthroscopic images during revision anterior cruciate ligament reconstruction of the patient illustrated in Figure 43-1. Significant malposition permitted bypass of the index femoral tunnel via endoscopic technique. (A) A guide pin is positioned at the site of the revision femoral tunnel. (B) Successful revision reconstruction with bypass of the index femoral tunnel.

revision reconstruction or whether it constitutes the problematic "near miss" that must be grafted because of its proximity to a more anatomically positioned tunnel.

We will typically obtain a non-arthrogram magnetic resonance imaging (MRI) scan as an adjunct for evaluating tunnel position as well as for identification of concomitant intra-articular pathology that may have contributed to failure of the index reconstruction. MRI permits evaluation of the intra-articular course of the graft and can be facilitated by capturing the plane parallel to the course of the graft.

Furthermore, we take care to evaluate not only the location of the femoral and tibial tunnels, but also to evaluate remaining bone stock and quality at each site—particularly when a soft-tissue graft has been used for the index reconstruction. We prefer computed tomography for qualitative and quantitative analysis of tunnel widening as radiographs.[6] Significant tunnel widening in combination with tunnel malposition, for example, can preclude alternate tunnel placement with a single procedure. Staged debridement with bone grafting may be required in these situations.

At the time of revision reconstruction, arthroscopic evaluation affords the final opportunity to evaluate tunnel position (Figure 43-2). After debridement of the failed graft, we look for the tibial tunnel to exit the plateau such that the center point of the graft lies along a line tangent with the posterior edge of the anterior horn of the lateral meniscus and 7 mm to 8 mm anterior to the anterior margin of the posterior cruciate ligament.[7] To evaluate the femoral tunnel we identify the over-the-top position and evaluate the proximity of the index tunnel to this point with respect to back-wall thickness and position along the lateral wall of the notch. Finally, we recommend the use of intraoperative fluoroscopy both during index reconstruction to prevent tunnel malposition and at the time of revision to ensure appropriate correction of tunnel malposition. Though some authors currently recommend the use of computer-assisted navigation techniques for more precise tunnel placement, we are unaware of any clinical data that would support the additional time and expense this technology demands.

References

1. Bealle D, Johnson DL. Technical pitfalls of anterior cruciate ligament surgery. *Clin Sports Med.* 1999;18(4):831-845, vi.
2. Allen CR, Giffin JR, Harner CD. Revision anterior cruciate ligament reconstruction. *Orthop Clin North Am.* 2003;34(1):79-98.
3. Yamamoto Y, Hsu WH, Woo SL, et al. Knee stability and graft function after anterior cruciate ligament reconstruction: a comparison of a lateral and an anatomical femoral tunnel placement. *Am J Sports Med.* 2004; 32(8):1825-1832.
4. Howell SH, Gittins ME, Gottlieb JE, et al. The relationship between the angle of the tibial tunnel in the coronal plane and loss of flexion and anterior laxity after anterior cruciate ligament reconstruction. *Am J Sports Med.* 2001;29(5):567-574.
5. Harner CD, Baek GH, Vogrin TM, et al. Quantitative analysis of human cruciate ligament insertions. *Arthroscopy.* 1999;15(7):741-749.
6. Webster KE, Feller JA, Elliott J, et al. A comparison of bone tunnel measurements made using computed tomography and digital plain radiography after anterior cruciate ligament reconstruction. *Arthroscopy.* 2004; 20(9):946-950.
7. Morgan CD, Kalman VR, Grawl DM. Definitive landmarks for reproducible tibial tunnel placement in anterior cruciate ligament reconstruction. *Arthroscopy.* 1995;11(3):275-288.

SECTION V

PEDIATRIC/ADOLESCENT QUESTIONS

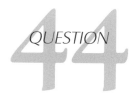
How Do You Manage the Adolescent With Open Growth Plates Who Has Sustained an ACL Injury?

Stephen F. Brockmeier, MD, and Riley J. Williams, III, MD

During recent years, increased attention has been given to the management of anterior cruciate ligament (ACL) injuries in the skeletally immature patient. Unfortunately, there is a paucity of peer-reviewed literature to guide the practitioner when confronted with this vexing problem. A variety of conservative and surgical approaches can be employed in this clinical circumstance. There is, however, no clear consensus on the indications for operative intervention or which method represents the "best" technique. What is clear is that the incidence of pediatric and adolescent ACL injuries is increasing.[1,2] Factors such as enhanced physician awareness, increased participation in high-risk pivoting sports by young people, and the application of sophisticated imaging methodologies such as magnetic resonance imaging (MRI) have all contributed to a more effective approach in detecting these ACL injuries.

The management of adolescent ACL injuries is controversial. Nonsurgical and surgical approaches both expose affected patients to real and theoretical risks. Conservative management of ACL insufficiency may result in meniscal injury and early joint degeneration. Of the surgery-associated risks, the most daunting is the potential for bony growth disturbance due to physeal injury. When surgery is considered, the risk factors for physeal injury include the use of large transphyseal tunnels, the placement of bone plugs or fixation devices that span the physis, and the use of an autograft patellar tendon graft (tibial bone plug harvested from the tibial tubercle). While a few reports of angular or longitudinal growth disturbances exist in the literature,[2,3] this complication is extremely uncommon.

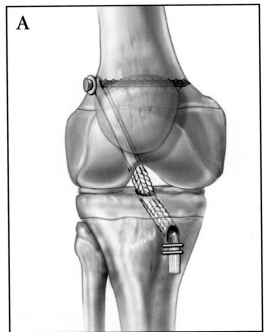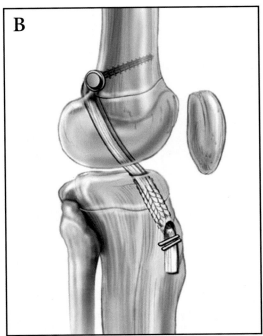

Figure 44-1. Authors' preferred technique for ACL reconstruction in a patient with open physes.

Many authors use the theoretical risk of physeal injury as a basis for applying a conservative management strategy until skeletal maturity is achieved. Extra-articular and nonanatomic ACL reconstructions have been described that avoid physeal violation for use in the pediatric ACL patient. Outcomes of these atypical types of ACL reconstruction have been unpredictable, with a high frequency of failure. Moreover, the literature has demonstrated an increased risk of intra-articular injuries (ie, medial meniscus tears) that are associated with nonsurgical management. In a series of skeletally immature patients with ACL ruptures, Graf reported that 7 of the 8 patients treated nonsurgically with a period of rehabilitation and bracing during activities experienced recurrent instability and sustained injuries to their medial meniscus.[4] Millett et al found that a delay in surgical ACL reconstruction of greater than 6 weeks was associated with a significant increase in the incidence of medial meniscal tears.[5] Woods and O'Connor noted no increase in the incidence of additional knee injuries in their series of 13 patients, but these authors stressed an absolute restriction of high-risk activities until physeal closure and eventual surgical reconstruction.[6] Practically speaking, this type of extreme activity modification is difficult to reliably employ in this patient population.

Because of the risk of recurrent knee instability and meniscal injury, we generally recommend a surgical approach to ACL injury in the skeletally immature patient. Our technique is an anatomic reconstruction that is similar to ACL reconstruction in the skeletally mature. However, this modified approach includes some alterations that minimize the potential insult to both the tibial and distal femoral growth plates (Figure 44-1). A soft-tissue graft is used for reconstruction (quadrupled hamstring) that utilizes both the gracilis and semitendinosis tendons. In adolescent patients, this graft is sufficient to stabilize the knee and is usually sized between 7 and 9 mm in diameter, depending on patient age and body habitus. A transphyseal tibial tunnel is used on the tibial side. After placing a guide pin in the ACL footprint, the tibial tunnel is created by power reaming only the anterior tibial cortex. The remainder of the tibial tunnel is then reamed by hand through the cancellous bone of proximal tibia. Hand reaming is done to avoid thermal injury to the tibial physis. For femoral fixation of the graft, an over-the-top approach is employed; no femoral tunnel is made. The cortical bone of the posterior-lateral femoral condyle and distal lateral femur is partially decorticated; fluoroscopy is used throughout to confirm that the distal femoral physis is avoided. The graft is fixed using a screw (post) and washer that is placed proximal to the growth plate. On the tibial side, the graft is typically fixed with a staple or soft-tissue button, depending on graft length.

The described approach offers a number of advantages. It is an anatomic ACL reconstruction, thus restoring relatively normal knee kinematics and limiting the risk of subsequent instability and meniscal injury. Patients may be able to resume their previous activities and sports. The risk of physeal arrest is extremely low because the only violation of a growth plate is a small diameter hole on the tibial side only that is filled with soft tissue. The femoral physis, which is more sensitive to physeal injury, is not disturbed. The senior author has used this technique in patients as young as 9 years of age and has anecdotally noted excellent patient outcomes with return to activity and no evidence of physeal disturbance or growth abnormality.

References

1. Shea KG, Pfeiffer R, Jo HW, et al. Anterior cruciate ligament injury in pediatric and adolescent soccer players: an analysis of insurance data. *J Pediatr Ortho*. 2004;24:623-628.
2. Kocher MS, Saxon HS, Hovis WD, et al. Management and complications of anterior cruciate ligament injuries in skeletally immature patients: survey of the Herodicus Society and the ACL Study Group. *J Pediatr Ortho*. 2002;22:452-457.
3. Koman JD, Sanders JO. Valgus deformity after reconstruction of the anterior cruciate ligament in a skeletally immature patient: a case report. *J Bone Joint Surg Am*. 1999;81:711-715.
4. Graf BK, Lange RH, Fujisaki CK, et al. Anterior cruciate ligament tears in skeletally immature patients: meniscal pathology at presentation and after attempted conservative treatment. *Arthroscopy*. 1992;8:229-233.
5. Millett PJ, Willis AA, Warren RF. Associated injuries in pediatric and adolescent anterior cruciate ligament injuries. *Arthroscopy*. 2002;18:955-959.
6. Woods GW, O'Connor DP. Delayed anterior cruciate ligament reconstruction in adolescents with open physes. *Am J Sports Med*. 2004;32:201-210.

WHAT SURGICAL OPTIONS ARE AVAILABLE IN THE ADOLESCENT WITH CONSIDERABLE GROWTH REMAINING?

Aimee S. Klapach, MD, and L. Pearce McCarty, III, MD

Optimal surgical management of complete anterior cruciate ligament (ACL) injury in skeletally immature patients with significant growth remaining continues to present a challenge. This management dilemma is underscored by a reported 11% incidence of growth disturbance following ACL reconstruction according to a recent survey of the Herodicus Society and ACL Study Group.[1]

The success of nonsurgical management, however, using prolonged bracing, physical therapy, and activity modification in the skeletally immature patient, is often poor with respect to return-to-sport and prevention of meniscal injury and concomitant pathology.[2,3] Kocher and colleagues reported a 31% rate of ACL reconstruction resulting from recurrent instability and reinjury in a group of predominantly skeletally immature patients with incomplete tears of the ACL treated nonoperatively.[4] Multivariate analysis identified partial tears of the posterolateral bundle of the ACL and tears measuring >50% of the ligament diameter (judged arthroscopically) to be independent predictors of subsequent reconstruction. Nevertheless, we have found functional bracing to represent a reasonable short-term (<6 months) management strategy in the rare individual in this population who is either low demand or proves capable of compliance with significant activity modification.

When considering surgical treatment of an adolescent with an ACL injury, we first determine the amount of growth remaining. This assessment is based upon chronological age, bone age (hand or pelvis), and secondary sex characteristics. Our treatment of patients with 6 months or less of growth remaining is identical to that of skeletally mature patients.

One should bear in mind the results of several studies when formulating an appropriate treatment plan. Stadelmaier and colleagues reported that 4 of 4 canines who underwent simple transphyseal drilling without soft-tissue graft interposition went on to at least partial epiphysiodesis, where as canines with soft-tissue graft interposition following drilling did not.[5] Of note, the grafts placed in this study were not tensioned.

Makela and colleagues drilled transphyseal tunnels in a rabbit model and observed no disturbance when the cross-sectional area of the defect was less than 3% of the total physeal area.[6] Osseous bridging was, however, demonstrated when the size of the defect was 7% or more of the total physeal cross-sectional area.

Edwards and colleagues performed ACL reconstruction using a transphyseal, tensioned soft-tissue graft with extraphyseal fixation in a canine model. They found significant femoral valgus deformity and significant tibial varus deformity without physeal bar formation.[7] A single degree of graft tensioning was used for all subject animals. Without an extraphyseal, tensioned graft control group, however, it is difficult to sort out the effects of transphyseal drilling versus graft tensioning on the growth disturbance observed.

Behr and colleagues conducted an anatomic study to determine the relationship between the over-the-top position and the distal femoral physis.[8] They found that the femoral attachment of the ACL was at an average of 3 mm from the level of the physis, and that the over-the-top position was at the level of the physis.

All of these studies have technical ramifications when contemplating ACL reconstruction in a skeletally immature population. Stadelmaier's findings suggest that soft-tissue grafts such as quadruple hamstring autograft are relatively safe from the standpoint of generating physeal disturbance. Makela's study indicates that more vertically oriented transphyseal tunnels, which disturb a smaller cross-sectional area of the physis, are preferred. Behr's relationship between the over-the-top position and the distal femoral physis cautions against reconstructive techniques that involve dissection or fixation at or near the over-the-top position. Finally, Edward's findings recommend against overtensioning of the graft, although it is difficult to quantify this recommendation.

Surgical options that minimize physeal risk for those patients who have significant growth remaining and who will not be compliant with functional bracing and activity modification include intra-articular, extraphyseal reconstruction, and hybrid techniques that typically utilize a transphyseal tunnel on the tibial side in combination with nonanatomic, over-the-top graft positioning on the femoral side.

Extra-articular procedures were performed in the past for ACL-deficient knees in adults. They were abandoned due to disappointing results. They hold appeal in the pediatric population because they avoid drilling across open physes. However, several long-term studies in the skeletally immature population have revealed recurrent pivoting leading to subsequent cartilage injury. We do not consider extra-articular procedures, therefore, to be adequate temporizing or definitive solutions.

Our preferred surgical technique for ACL reconstruction in the skeletally immature with significant growth remaining is a 2-incision, combination procedure that utilizes a small diameter (6 or 7 mm), vertically oriented, transphyseal tibial tunnel in combination with an over-the-top position on the femur, similar to that originally described by Andrews and Noyes (Figure 45-1).[9] Our graft of choice is double-looped semitendinosus-gracilis autograft. Fixation is achieved on both the femoral and tibial sides via a "double-staple" technique, in which the graft is fixed with one staple then folded back onto itself and fixed with a second staple. The folded portion of the graft is then sutured to itself with a running whipstitch using a braided, nonabsorbable suture. We utilize intraoperative fluoroscopy to ensure that femoral and tibial fixation is proximal and distal to the physes respectively. A standard soft-tissue ACL rehab protocol is prescribed postoperatively with return to unrestricted activity at 4 to 6 months.

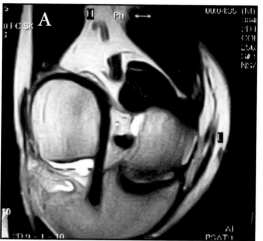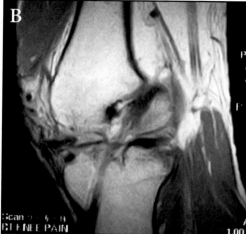

Figure 45-1. Postoperative magnetic resonance imaging (MRI) illustrating graft position in hybrid technique. (A) Three-year postoperative coronal MRI image demonstrating femoral over-the-top position of graft. (B) Sagittal MRI image demonstrating transtibial tunnel. The patient's physes are closed.

References

1. Kocher MS, Saxon HS, Hovis WD, Hawkins RJ. Management and complications of anterior cruciate ligament injuries in skeletally immature patients: survey of the Herodicus Society and the ACL Study Group. *J Pediatr Orthop.* 2002;22(4):452-457.
2. Millett PJ, Willis AA, Warren RF. Associated injuries in pediatric and adolescent anterior cruciate ligament tears: does a delay in treatment increase the risk of meniscal tear? *Arthroscopy.* 2002;18(9):955-959.
3. Woods GW, O'Connor DP. Delayed anterior cruciate ligament reconstruction in adolescents with open physes. *Am J Sports Med.* 2004;32(1):201-210.
4. Kocher MS, Micheli LJ, Zurakowski D, Luke A. Partial tears of the anterior cruciate ligament in children and adolescents. *Am J Sports Med.* 2002;30(5):697-703.
5. Stadelmaier DM, Arnoczky SP, Dodds J, Ross H. The effect of drilling and soft tissue grafting across open growth plates. A histologic study. *Am J Sports Med.* 1995;23(4):431-435.
6. Makela EA, Vainionpaa S, Vihtonen K, Mero M, Rokkanen P. The effect of trauma to the lower femoral epiphyseal plate. An experimental study in rabbits. *J Bone Joint Surg Br.* 1988;70(2):187-191.
7. Edwards TB, Greene CC, Baratta RV, Zieske A, Willis RB. The effect of placing a tensioned graft across open growth plates. A gross and histologic analysis. *J Bone Joint Surg Am.* 2001;83-A(5):725-734.
8. Behr CT, Potter HG, Paletta GA Jr. The relationship of the femoral origin of the anterior cruciate ligament and the distal femoral physeal plate in the skeletally immature knee. An anatomic study. *Am J Sports Med.* 2001;29(6):781-787.
9. Andrews M, Noyes FR, Barber-Westin SD. Anterior cruciate ligament allograft reconstruction in the skeletally immature athlete. *Am J Sports Med.* 1994;22(1):48-54.

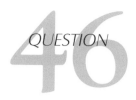

My Daughter Is a High School Basketball Athlete

What Are the Risks of Tearing Her ACL? If She Has That Knee Fixed, What Are the Risks for the Opposite Knee? Are There ACL Injury Prevention Programs Available?

Nicholas T. Dutchenshen, MD, and Thomas J. Gill, MD

Anterior cruciate ligament (ACL) injury occurs with a 4-fold to 6-fold greater incidence in female athletes compared to male athletes playing the same cutting and landing sports.[1] Injury rates vary according to sex, sport played, and level of participation. There have been several studies that have examined differences between genders that may account for an increased incidence of ACL tears in women. In part, this research has lead to successful training programs that aim to decrease the number of ACL tears in female athletes.

For females playing high school basketball, the overall injury rate per 100 players is 28.7, with 15.7% of these injuries occurring in the knee (4.5 injuries per 100 players).[2] Rebounding in practice is the most frequently reported activity during injury. A recent study suggests that patients who rupture their ACL have a 6.4% chance of rerupturing their reconstructed ACL graft and a 5.7% chance of rupturing the ACL on their opposite knee within 5 years. In other words, the risk of suffering an ACL tear to either the reconstructed knee or the contralateral knee is nearly identical.[3] Other authors have shown that athletes returning to sports that specifically involve cutting and pivoting are more likely to rupture their contralateral ACL rather than their reconstructed ACL.[3,4]

Why do female athletes have a higher incidence of ACL tears than males? The mechanism underlying the gender disparity is likely multifactorial. Several theories have been proposed, and they include anatomical, hormonal, and neuromuscular differences between genders.

Numerous anatomic distinctions have been observed between male and female athletes. The differences include the presence of the following in females: a wider pelvis, increased Q angle, smaller notch width, smaller ACL, increased generalized joint laxity, increased hamstring flexibility, increased anterior tibial translation, and increased foot pronation/navicular drop.[5] However, no one anatomical risk factor has been directly and independently correlated to an increase in noncontact ACL injury.

Numerous studies have examined the effect of hormones on ACL tears. It has been shown that estrogen can affect the tensile properties of ligaments and estrogen receptors are present in female ACL fibroblasts. Moreover, estrogen has been shown to alter neuromuscular function in both the central and peripheral nervous system.[5] As with the anatomical differences between sexes, it seems that the literature has an equal number of researchers who agree and disagree as to the effect of hormones on the incidence of ACL tears.

More recently, neuromuscular differences between men and women have been examined in order to explain the difference in the incidence of ACL tears. Wojtys demonstrated that women exhibit less muscular protection of the knee ligaments with the tibia in internal rotation than men.[6] Perhaps the most important finding to date is the precision with which males and females are able to decelerate from landing and control dynamic valgus and tibial translation. This is thought to be the result of a discrepancy in the balance between hamstring-to-quadriceps strength and recruitment. Thus, when a female lands from a jump she is more prone to hyperextend her knee and suffer a noncontact ACL injury.

The latest research on neuromuscular control and the differences that exist between men and women have led to programs aimed at ACL injury prevention. Neuromuscular and proprioceptive training in female athletes has been shown to increase active knee stabilization in the laboratory and decrease the incidence of ACL injury.[7] There are a number of successful training programs that teach female athletes how to actively recruit muscles that decrease joint motion and protect the ACL during athletic activity, primarily landing from a jump. A recent study by Mandelbaum showed that a neuromuscular and proprioceptive training program was effective in decreasing the number of ACL tears in women by an average of 81% over a period of 2 years.[8]

There are many programs whose goals are to prevent injury to the ACL. The program described by Mandelbaum, PEP (Prevent Injury and Enhance Performance), shares numerous similarities with other preventative programs.[8] Athletes watch a videotape and are instructed to perform several stretching and strengthening exercises for their trunk and lower extremity as well as a number of plyometric and agility drills during their routine warm-up. Most importantly, this program emphasizes proper cutting and landing techniques. This includes engaging hip and knee flexion, avoiding genu valgum at the knee on landing and lateral maneuvers, and addressing proper deceleration techniques. The program also employs strengthening the hip abductors and hamstrings.

The incidence of injury to the ACL is currently more common in women than men. There are many anatomical, hormonal, and neuromuscular differences between the 2 sexes that may account for this discrepancy. However, with continuing research and more attention to programs that promote neuromuscular and proprioceptive training, we may begin to see fewer ACL tears in the female athlete.

References

1. Arendt E, Dick R. Knee injury patterns among men and women in collegiate basketball and soccer: NCAA data and review of literature. *Am J Sports Med.* 1995;23:694-701.
2. Powell JW, Kim D, Barber-Foss. Sex-related injury patterns among selected high school sports. *Am J Sports Med.* 2000;28:385-391.
3. Salmon LB, Russell VB, Musgrove TM, et al. Incidence and risk factors for graft rupture and contralateral rupture after anterior cruciate ligament reconstruction. *Arthroscopy.* 2005;21(8):948-957.
4. Shelbourne K, Davis T, Klootwyk T. The relationship between intercondylar notch width of the femur and the incidence of anterior cruciate ligament tears. *Am J Sports Med.* 1998;26:402-408.
5. Hewett TE, Myer GD, Ford KR. Anterior cruciate ligament injuries in female athletes: part 1, mechanisms and risk factors. *Am J Sports Med.* 2006;34:299-311.
6. Wojtys EM, Huston LJ, Schock HJ, Boylan JP, Ashton-Miller JA. Gender differences in muscular protection of the knee in torsion in size-matched athletes. *J Bone Joint Surg Am.* 2003;85:782-789.
7. Hewett TE, Lindenfeld TN, Riccobene JV, Noyes FR. The effect of neuromuscular training on the incidence of knee injury in female athletes: a prospective study. *Am J Sports Med.* 1999;27:699-706.
8. Mandelbaum BR, Silvers HJ, Watanabe JF, et al. Effectiveness of a neuromuscular and proprioceptive training program in preventing anterior cruciate ligament injuries in female athletes: 2-year follow-up. *Am J Sports Med.* 2005;33:1103-1010.

SECTION VI

MISCELLANEOUS QUESTIONS

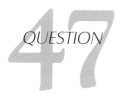

WHAT IS YOUR PREFERRED NONOPERATIVE TREATMENT PROTOCOL FOR ACUTE ACL INJURIES IN PATIENTS WHO DO NOT WISH TO UNDERGO SURGERY?

Kyle R. Flik, MD

Nonoperative treatment for anterior cruciate ligament (ACL) rupture has not been a successful option for patients who participate in high-level activities, especially sports that involve cutting or pivoting maneuvers.[1] Nonetheless, some patients choose to avoid surgery, at least in the short term. For example, the athlete with limited eligibility or the one who must compete to demonstrate scholarship worthiness may elect to avoid surgery. In this section I will describe the ideal candidate for nonoperative treatment and will outline important rehabilitation guidelines to optimize nonsurgical outcome in the ACL-deficient patient.

Nonoperative treatment is most likely to be successful if the appropriate candidate is identified early after injury and appropriate rehabilitation is begun. The best candidate for nonoperative treatment has an isolated ACL injury (no meniscus or concomitant ligamentous injury) and no recurrent episodes of giving way. I am most comfortable treating this patient nonoperatively if he has demonstrated that he has no pain in the knee, no recurrent effusions, and no giving-way sensations. In this setting, anti-inflammatory medications combined with an early physical therapy protocol and use of an ACL brace may be an appropriate management strategy. Patients with injury to other knee ligaments or repairable meniscus damage in addition to the torn ACL do poorly with nonoperative management. After ruling concomitant injury out, I will start a patient immediately on a physical therapy program geared toward maximizing the patient's chances for successful return to high-level sports without recurrent instability.

Important components to a successful physical therapy program for the ACL-injured patient include lower extremity muscular strength and endurance exercises, knee joint mobility exercises, agility and sport-specific training, and perturbation training techniques. Perturbation training involves the application of destabilizing forces to the patient's involved limb while the patient stands on tilt boards and roller boards. In a study by Fitzgerald et al, patients who underwent additional perturbation training had a significantly higher success rate of returning to high-level activity without ACL reconstruction surgery.[2]

The first goal in therapy is to regain painless range of motion and to control postinjury swelling. Cryotherapy and oral anti-inflammatory medication are mainstays of early postinjury treatment. Quadriceps femoris weakness is of great concern following ACL injury and has been shown to correlate with poor outcome.[3] Quadriceps weakness should therefore be resolved early in the rehabilitation course, with the use of electrical stimulation if needed. Resisted leg extensions in a limited range of 90 to 45 degrees of flexion are performed, since in this range there is no significant anterior shear force on the tibiofemoral joint. Hamstring strengthening is also emphasized, primarily with the use of resisted leg curls. Other lower extremity strength exercises such as leg press and squat lifts can be performed safely in a limited range of 0 to 45 degrees of flexion.

Cardiovascular endurance training is selected to best reflect the patient's sport or work environment. For example, runners may begin a graded running program, or cyclists may initiate endurance training with stationary cycling. When the activity is comfortably performed for short periods without pain or swelling, the duration and intensity are increased.

Agility training is an important component of the rehabilitation process. This allows patients to adapt to quick changes in direction. A functional knee brace is used. Sport-specific drills are combined with agility exercises once full-speed agility exercises are tolerated without pain, swelling, or apprehension.

The perturbation program involves the application of translational perturbations to the involved limb through a roller board or tilt board. Balance is developed during this mode of rehabilitation.

Despite successful reports of return to high-level athletic endeavors in some patients after nonoperative treatment of acute ACL injury, I still advise my patients to avoid cutting and pivoting activities if possible if they choose a nonoperative course of treatment.

References

1. Barrack RL, Bruckner JD, Kneisl J, Inman WS, Alexander AH. The outcome of nonoperatively treated complete tears of the anterior cruciate ligament in active young adults. *Clin Orthop Relat Res*. 1990;259:192-199.
2. Fitzgerald GK, Axe MJ, Snyder-Mackler L. Proposed practice guidelines for nonoperative anterior cruciate ligament rehabilitation of physically active individuals. *J Orthop Sports Phys Ther*. 2000;30(4):194-203.
3. Lephart SM, Perrin DH, Fu FH. Relationship between selected physical characteristics and functional capacity in the anterior cruciate ligament-insufficient athlete. *J Orthop Sports Phys Ther*. 1992;16:174-181.

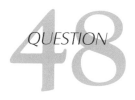

WHAT ARE THE LONG-TERM IMPLICATIONS OF THE PATIENT WITH RECURRENT INSTABILITY IN THE SETTING OF UNTREATED ACL INJURIES?

Scott A. Rodeo, MD

Some patients with anterior cruciate ligament (ACL) tears will not develop recurrent instability and can be treated conservatively. These patients have been termed *copers*. Unfortunately, there is no way to accurately predict which patients may fall into this small group. The majority of active patients with an untreated ACL tear will experience recurrent instability. Recurrent episodes of instability can lead to three detrimental changes in the knee: (1) meniscus injury, (2) articular cartilage injury, and (3) progressive knee instability. I will discuss each of these in turn.

The primary risk associated with instability episodes is meniscus tear. There is an increased risk of medial meniscus tears in knees with chronic ACL insufficiency. Basic laboratory studies demonstrate a biomechanical interdependence between the medial meniscus and the ACL. This interdependence means that there are increased forces on the medial meniscus in the ACL-insufficient knee, which explains the propensity for medial meniscus tears.[1] Vertical longitudinal tears of the medial meniscus are more common in the ACL-insufficient knee. This tear pattern may be repairable, and aggressive attempts should be made to preserve the meniscus.

Most meniscus tears are not repairable, however, and will require partial meniscectomy. It is well established that meniscus loss increases the risk of progressive arthrosis. There is a progressive increase in articular contact stress and a decrease in contact area following meniscectomy that is directly proportional to the degree of meniscus loss.[2] In my opinion, one of the primary reasons for ACL reconstruction is meniscus preservation.

Loss of the medial meniscus may also compromise later ACL reconstruction. The biomechanical interdependence between the ACL and the medial meniscus produces increased forces on the ACL in the medial meniscus-deficient knee. Clinical results support this data, as there are inferior results (using KT-1000 arthrometry) following ACL reconstruction in knees that have had prior medial meniscectomy compared to knees with an intact medial meniscus.[3] In fact, medial meniscus transplantation in conjunction with ACL reconstruction can be considered if there has been prior subtotal medial meniscectomy and if other indications are met. The rationale for meniscus transplantation in this setting is to protect the ACL graft, in addition to the role of the meniscus in load transmission.

Recurrent instability episodes also increase the risk of articular cartilage injury. Chondral surface injury can occur in both medial and lateral compartments and often occurs with concomitant meniscus injury. Clinical studies of the outcome of ACL reconstruction clearly demonstrate inferior results in knees with articular cartilage injury.[4] At the present time there is no data to conclusively demonstrate that ACL reconstruction decreases the risk of later chondral injury or the development of arthritis; however, meniscal preservation will decrease the risk of progressive joint degeneration.

Lastly, recurrent instability episodes can also lead to progressive increases in joint laxity. Such an increase in laxity is attributed to changes ("stretching out") in secondary stabilizers, which are overloaded in the ACL-insufficient knee. For example, the medial collateral ligament is a secondary stabilizer in the ACL-insufficient knee (similar to the medial meniscus, as discussed above) and thus may become more lax over time in the ACL-insufficient knee.[5] Prior studies have shown increased total anterior-posterior laxity in knees with chronic ACL instability compared to acute ACL injury. It may be more difficult to stabilize such knees with increased preoperative laxity.

References

1. Papageorgiou CD, Gil JE, Kanamori A, Fenwick JA, Woo SL, Fu FH. The biomechanical interdependence between the anterior cruciate ligament replacement graft and the medial meniscus. *Am J Sports Med*. 2001; 29(2):226-231.
2. Lee SJ, Aadalen KJ, Malaviya P, et al. Tibiofemoral contact mechanics after serial medial meniscectomies in the human cadaveric knee. *Am J Sports Med*. 2006;34(8):1334-1344.
3. Shelbourne KD, Gray T. Results of anterior cruciate ligament reconstruction based on meniscus and articular cartilage status at the time of surgery. Five- to fifteen-year evaluations. *Am J Sports Med*. 2000;28(4):446-452.
4. Noyes FR, Barber-Westin SD, Roberts CS. Use of allografts after failed treatment of rupture of the anterior cruciate ligament. *J Bone Joint Surg Am*. 1994;76(7):1019-1031.
5. Sullivan D, Levy IM, Sheskier S, Torzilli PA, Warren RF. Medial restraints to anterior-posterior motion of the knee. *J Bone Joint Surg Am*. 1984;66(6):930-936.

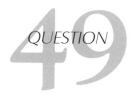

WHAT IMPLICATIONS DOES ACL RECONSTRUCTION HAVE ON THE FUTURE DEVELOPMENT OF DEGENERATIVE ARTHRITIS?

Kurt P. Spindler, MD, and James L. Carey, MD

The causes of degenerative joint disease in the post-traumatic knee are multifactorial and include the following: articular impaction with initial trauma, meniscal injury, operative trauma, and abnormal knee kinematics.

Articular impaction of the lateral femoral condyle by the posterolateral tibial plateau may occur at the time of anterior cruciate ligament (ACL) rupture when the tibia subluxes anteriorly with some internal rotation. The archetypal bone bruising pattern associated with this impaction is best visualized on the sagittal images of the knee as increased T2 signal in the region of the sulcus terminalis of the lateral femoral condyle and the posterolateral tibial plateau. A recent review of the literature on the natural history of these bone bruises concluded that this blunt injury to the articular cartilage and subchondral bone can alter articular cartilage homeostasis and induce early degenerative changes.[1]

Injury to the meniscus (Figure 49-1) occurs in approximately 25% of ACL ruptures. A literature review that examined the frequency of post-traumatic knee degenerative joint disease found a number of retrospective studies with follow-up times between 5 and 20 years.[2] These authors concluded that 50% to 70% of patients with an ACL rupture combined with meniscus tear have some radiographic changes after 15 to 20 years.[2] Further, one study of 53 patients at 7 years post–ACL reconstruction found that acute ACL reconstruction with meniscal preservation was shown to have the lowest incidence of radiographic evidence of degenerative changes.[3]

The goal of ACL reconstruction is to restore stability in order to prevent future subluxation events, preserve the meniscus, and minimize further degenerative changes. However, the operative trauma of ACL reconstruction may contribute to the development

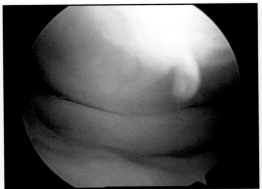

Figure 49-1. A bucket-handle meniscal tear is often associated with ACL rupture, as in this case.

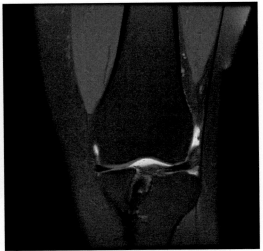

Figure 49-2. Standard tunnels required for graft passage are approximately 10 mm in diameter initially and may dilate further with time. These tunnels may alter the bony architecture that supports the joint surfaces similar to a mattress with an inadequate foundation (box spring).

of degenerative joint disease. The procedure commonly results in a hemarthrosis. Rare postoperative complications of knee sepsis and arthrofibrosis probably increase the risk for knee arthritis as well. Further, the tunnels required for graft passage (Figure 49-2) subtly alter the bony architecture that supports the joint surfaces.

Tearing or rupturing your ACL alters the normal mechanics (kinematics) of the knee. Even the most successful ACL reconstructions do not restore normal knee kinematics. Abnormal knee kinematics accelerate the normal wear of the articular surfaces.

The exact contribution of each injury, patient characteristics, and activity demands on the knee are not known but are being investigated by multicenter prospective longitudinal studies.

References

1. Nakamae A, Bahr R, Krosshaug T. Natural history of bone bruises after acute knee injury: clinical outcome and histopathological findings. *Knee Surg Sports Traumatol Arthrosc.* 2006;14:1252-1258.
2. Gillquist J, Messner K. Anterior cruciate ligament reconstruction and the long term incidence of gonarthrosis. *Sports Med.* 1999;27:143-156.
3. Jomha NM, Borton DC, Clingeleffer AJ, Pinczewski LA. Long term osteoarthritic changes in anterior cruciate ligament reconstructed knees. *Clin Orthop Relat Res.* 1999;358:188-193.

Printed in the United States
by Baker & Taylor Publisher Services